Peru

Improving Health Care for the Poor

The World Bank
Washington, D.C.

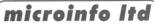

Library of Congress Cataloging-in-Publication Data has been applied for.

CONTENTS

TABLES

DIAGRAMS

BOXES

ABSTRACT

The Peruvian health sector –measured in terms of spending, infrastructure and use– has recovered rapidly after collapsing in the late 1980s and early 1990s as a result of hyperinflation and terrorism. Infant mortality and child malnutrition have also improved rapidly in recent years. Despite these improvements in both inputs and outcomes, policy-makers face three key challenges and concerns. First, how to continue to reduce the large gap between the health status of the poor and that of the non-poor. Second, how to increase the resources assigned to provide care for the poor. Third, how to increase the efficiency in the use of these resources. Several reforms have been tried during the years of recuperation of the sector in response to those challenges. The most successful in the area of health provision consisted of building large targeted programs to support primary care by allocating health workers based on regional priorities set by a poverty map, and by assigning funds for nutrition and to combat the diseases of the poor. In some areas there has also been a program to transfer the provision of primary health services to the communities with public funding and a contract defining the targets to be met. In the area of health financing, new payment systems are under implementation for schoolchildren and under development for mothers and younger children. This report is produced as an input to be used by the Government to continue to develop its agenda to improve health care for the poor. A leitmotif that emerges from this report and is reflected in its conclusions and recommendations is that much can be gained by sustaining and deepening the reforms directed toward improving health care for the poor. For that to happen, key outstanding issues in providing, financing, managing, and manning health services have to be resolved. These key issues are discussed in the report and recommendations are made for dealing with them.

PREFACE AND ACKNOWLEDGMENTS

Recent developments in Peru's health sector have been extraordinary. Since the early 1990s, both health care and health care expenditure have multiplied, with increased emphasis being given to primary care and improved access to services in poor rural and urban areas. Concurrently there has been enormous institutional innovation in the sector. Many new programs have been implemented, and many more new ideas have been proposed. This report was requested by the Government as an instrument to help it grasp where the sector stands today and what the priorities for the future should be. Its twin objectives are: (i) to help the government's efforts to formulate a strategy to continue to improve the health outcomes of the poor; and (ii) to guide World Bank and other development agency activities to help implement such a strategy.

The report was prepared by the World Bank as a contribution to its ongoing policy dialogue with the Government of Peru. It is based on the findings of a World Bank mission that visited Peru in April 1998 and on numerous reports prepared during the last two years by our colleagues at the Ministry of Health. The mission members who wrote contributions were: Daniel Cotlear (task team leader and main author of this report), Mari Sol Concha (epidemiology and service provision), Tarcisio Castañeda (targeting and community participation), and Richard Webb (labor markets and primary care). Cuanto S.A. processed the survey data used in the report. The initial report was updated, based on numerous discussions held in 1998 and 1999 with officials from the Ministry of Health and the Ministry of Finance as well as interviews with members of universities, research centers and nongovernmental organizations. Laura Altobelli (public health specialist) and Jonathan Cavanagh (editor) contributed to the final version, which was patiently desktop-edited by Patricia Bernedo.

The study was initiated while the Minister of Health was Marino Costa and was concluded while the Minister was Alejandro Aguinaga. Both of them, their key advisors and many officials and consultants were extremely helpful to the preparation of the study. Special thanks go to Augusto Meloni who helped us understand the sector and its issues through many hours of discussion and to Carlos Bardales, Danilo Fernandez, Pedro Francke, Ariel Frisancho, Alvaro Gaillour, Diego Gonzalez, Jaime Johnson, Ulises Jorge, Doris Lituma, Luis Manrique, Pedro Mendoza, Percy Minaya, Margarita Petrera, Nina Sotomarino, Raul Torres, Victor Zamora y Eduardo Zárate.

Comments and guidance were received at the Bank from Evangeline Javier, who contributed to the report at all stages of the process and from Charles Griffin, Livia Benavides, Alex Precker, Davidson Gwatkins, Christopher Lovelace and Ernesto May. Silvia Raw and Amanda Glassman from the IDB and Luis Seminario from USAID provided useful comments. In Peru, the final draft report was discussed in April 1999 with the top authorities of the Ministry of Health, the regional health directors, officials from the Ministry of Finance, the Health Commission of the National Congress, academics, NGOs and donors.

ACRONYMS AND ABBREVIATIONS

ANC	Ante-Natal Care
ARI	Acute Respiratory Infections
BCG	Vaccine against Tuberculosis
CISRESA	Infrastructure Census *(Censo de Infraestructura Sanitaria y Recursos del Sector Salud)*
CLAS	Community-managed Publicly Financed Health Committee *(Comité Local de Administración de Salud)*
DALY	Disability-Adjusted Life Year
DPT	Vaccine against Diphteria, Pertussis and Tetanus
DGSP	Office of the Director General of Health
DIGESA	Office of the Director General of Environmental Health *(Dirección General de Salud Ambiental)*
ENDES	Demographic and Health Survey *(Encuesta de Demografía y Salud)*
ENNIV	Living Standards Measurement Survey *(Encuesta de Niveles de Vida)*
ESAN	Graduate Business School *(Escuela Superior de Administración de Negocios)*
ESSALUD	New name for IPSS
HIS	Health Information System
IDB	Inter-American Development Bank
IEC	Information, Education, and Communication
IMR	Infant Mortality Rate
INS	National Health Institute *(Instituto Nacional de Salud)*
PPF	Project Preparation Facility
IPSS	Peruvian Social Security Institute *(Instituto Peruano de Seguridad Social)*
LAC	Latin America and the Caribbean
LHP	Local Health Plans
LSMS	Living Standards Measurement Survey
MCH	Maternal and Child Health
MEF	Ministry of Economy and Finance *(Ministerio de Economía y Finanzas)*
MINPRE	Ministry of the Presidency *(Ministerio de la Presidencia)*
MINSA	Ministry of Health *(Ministerio de Salud)*
MCH	Maternal-Child Insurance *(Seguro Materno Infantil)*
NGO	Nongovernmental Organizations
OGP	MINSA's Planning Office *(Oficina General de Planificación)*
ORT	Oral Rehydration Therapy
FONCODES	Social Investment Fund *(Fondo de Compensación y Desarrollo Social)*
PACFO	Complementary Food Program
PAHO	Pan American Health Organization
PFSS	Strengthening Health Services Project *(Proyecto de Fortalecimiento de los Servicios de Salud)*
PHC	Primary Health Clinics
PSBPT	Basic Health for All Program *(Programa de Salud Básica para Todos)*
PSMU	Public Sector Modernization Unit *(Unidad Coordinadora de Modernización del Sub-sector Público de Salud)*
PSNB	Health and Basic Nutrition Project *(Proyecto de Salud y Nutrición Básica)*
REDES	Health Networks
SE	Insurance for schoolchildren *(Seguro Escolar)*
SERUM	Intern Service in Rural and Urban Marginal Areas *(Servicio Rural y Urbano Marginal)*
SMI	Maternal-Child Insurance *(Seguro Materno Infantil)*
UNICEF	United Nations Children's Fund
UNFPA	United Nations Fund for Population Activities
USAID	United States Agency for International Development
WHO	World Health Organization

Government Fiscal Year
January 1- December 31

Currency Equivalents
Currency Unit= Soles

Vice President:	Shahid Javed Burki
Country Director:	Isabel Guerrero
Sector Director:	Xavier Coll
Sector Specialist:	Charles Griffin
Task Manager:	Daniel Cotlear

Resumen Ejecutivo e Introducción

El sector de salud peruano se ha recuperado rápidamente tras el colapso ocurrido entre fines de la década del 80 y comienzos de los años 90 como resultado de la hiperinflación y el terrorismo. Esta recuperación ha sido acompañada por importantes reformas en los servicios de atención primaria del Ministerio de Salud (MINSA) y ha contribuido a una mejora significativa en la salud de la población. Este estudio evalúa las principales reformas en atención primaria introducidas por el MINSA y hace recomendaciones para continuar mejorando la atención de salud para los grupos de menores ingresos.

El gasto público y privado total en el área de salud aumentó en términos reales en más del 50% en los tres años posteriores a 1994. La oferta de servicios de salud aumentó de manera pronunciada, particularmente en la atención primaria de salud: el número de clínicas de salud primaria aumentó en dos tercios y se extendió su horario de atención. Hubo también un aumento del 55% en los puestos de empleo para profesionales de salud, mayormente en atención primaria. La demanda de servicios también se incrementó. En el ámbito nacional, el uso de servicios creció en 59% en sólo tres años. En las zonas rurales, se vio un crecimiento similar al promedio nacional. Los indicadores de salud también han mejorado rápidamente en los últimos años. Esto ha estado asociado a la mejora en los ingresos y las condiciones de vida y a la expansión de servicios de salud. La mortalidad infantil y la desnutrición infantil, por ejemplo, disminuyeron en aproximadamente un 30% durante la segunda mitad de la década y es probable que hayan continuado mejorando desde entonces. Pese a estas mejoras tanto en los recursos como en los resultados, los encargados de formular las políticas de salud enfrentan todavía tres desafíos y preocupaciones fundamentales.

En primer lugar, cómo continuar *reduciendo la brecha entre el nivel de salud de los pobres y el de los otros grupos*. El Perú sigue siendo un caso atípico en América Latina, puesto que a pesar de las mejoras recientes, todavía exhibe un índice de mortalidad infantil muy alto para un país con su nivel de ingresos. Los altos índices de mortalidad infantil se concentran en la población pobre, mientras que los indicadores de los grupos de mayores ingresos se aproximan más al promedio latinoamericano. La población pobre, dividida entre las zonas rurales y urbanas, es más vulnerable a la mala salud debido a una combinación de bajo nivel educativo, condiciones ambientales insalubres y acceso limitado a los servicios de salud. Los pobres se encuentran más expuestos que el resto de la población a las enfermedades transmisibles, muchas de ellas exacerbadas por problemas ambientales, tales como instalaciones sanitarias deficientes y transmisión vectorial. Aunque el acceso a servicios primarios para niños de más de un mes de edad ha mejorado enormemente en los últimos años, los pobres continúan sufriendo por la falta de acceso a servicios para madres y para recién nacidos, quienes requieren servicios de atención primaria y también prestados en hospitales.

En segundo lugar, cómo *incrementar los recursos asignados a la atención de salud de la población pobre*. El Perú, a pesar del incremento de años recientes, todavía sigue asignando menos recursos a la salud que la mayoría de sus vecinos. La proporción del

PIB asignada al sector de salud, 4.1% en 1997, equivale a unos dos tercios del promedio latinoamericano. La disponibilidad de médicos, 10 por cada 10,000 habitantes, representa sólo un 70% del promedio latinoamericano. También existe gran desigualdad en el consumo de bienes y de servicios de salud. El consumo per cápita de bienes y servicios de salud es aproximadamente 4.5 veces mayor entre el 20% del nivel socioeconómico más alto que en el 20% del nivel más bajo. Aunque gran parte de esta diferencia se debe al mayor gasto privado en atención médica por los grupos de mayores ingresos, dicha diferencia se ve sólo parcialmente compensada por el Ministerio de Salud (MINSA), el cual teóricamente debería servir a los sectores pobres, pero en la práctica asigna a los pobres sumas similares a las asignadas a los otros grupos.

El tercer desafío es *cómo utilizar más eficientemente estos recursos.* El gasto total en la salud asciende a aproximadamente US$2,700 millones al año, divididos en partes iguales entre los sectores privado y público (véase la casilla 1). Aproximadamente la mitad del gasto público se canaliza a través del MINSA, el cual asigna un poco menos de la mitad de sus recursos a la atención primaria de salud. El sistema sufre de importantes deficiencias, reflejadas en la coexistencia de una gran capacidad subutilizada en todos los subsectores, con necesidades insatisfechas y congestión de algunos servicios. Las ineficiencias más importantes se deben a la fragmentación, la ausencia de competencia y la ausencia de separación entre el financiamiento y la provisión. También existen deficiencias significativas en los centros y puestos de atención primaria (CPAPS), reflejadas en baja productividad y una adecuación insuficiente a las necesidades locales.

Casilla 1. La estructura del sector de salud

El sistema de salud peruano es una amalgama compleja de varios programas públicos y un sector privado amplio, cada uno de los cuales es simultáneamente proveedor y financiador de servicios. Cada subsector sigue un curso independiente; existe poca coordinación y casi ninguna competencia entre proveedores o entre financiadores de servicios. Los programas públicos principales son: (i) el Ministerio de Salud (MINSA), financiado por recaudaciones tributarias y pagos directos de los usuarios, que en teoría presta servicios a los sectores pobres, y (ii) el ESSALUD (anteriormente Instituto Peruano de Seguridad Social -- IPSS), financiado por un impuesto del 9% sobre planillas de sueldos, que en teoría cubre todas las necesidades de atención médica de sus contribuyentes los cuales son mayormente trabajadores del sector formal de la economía. El sector privado se financia casi en su totalidad por pagos en efectivo de los pacientes y sus familias, ya que la cobertura de los seguros privados es muy reducida y los programas públicos (con muy pocas excepciones) no contratan servicios de proveedores privados.

Según encuestas de hogares, el MINSA desempeña un papel importante en la prestación de servicios clínicos, ya que presta dos tercios de los servicios de hospitalización y 44% de las consultas ambulatorias. El sector privado también es muy importante como proveedor de servicios ambulatorios, tanto en zonas urbanas como rurales, y también para los pobres. El IPSS, que constituye el 25% del gasto nacional en la salud, presta 18% de los servicios ambulatorios y 23% de los servicios de hospitalización, concentrándose estos servicios en las ciudades principales y exclusivamente en beneficio de la población con recursos.

Se realizó un análisis de la incidencia de beneficios a fin de entender la función de los diversos subsectores en la atención de los pobres. El consumo de la atención médica es una combinación de un elemento privado con el gasto canalizado a través del MINSA y el IPSS. La mayor parte de la desigualdad en el consumo de servicios de salud resulta de la desigualdad en el ingreso, pues los grupos de mayores ingresos pueden destinar más recursos privados a la atención médica que los pobres. El IPSS contribuye a esta situación al atender únicamente a los empleados del sector formal y sus familias, quienes están concentrados en los niveles más altos de la distribución de ingresos. El gasto de MINSA se distribuye por igual entre ricos y pobres.

Se ha intentado varias reformas durante los años de recuperación del sector. Algunas estan rindiendo fruto, otras fracasaron. Hubo varios intentos fallidos de impulsar reformas extensas en el sector, con el propósito de superar las grandes ineficiencias creadas por la fragmentación y la ausencia de competencia.[1] La innovación que alcanzó el mayor éxito consistió en la creación de extensos programas focalizados. Estos apoyan la atención primaria mediante el financiamiento de trabajadores de salud asignados a zonas seleccionadas con el uso de un mapa de pobreza, y mediante la asignación de fondos para la nutrición y la lucha contra las enfermedades que afligen a los pobres. En algunas zonas, los programas focalizados han servido para experimentar con formas de organización que incentivan lograr la participación de la comunidad.[2]

Este informe se ha elaborado con el objetivo de servir como insumo para que el gobierno continúe desarrollando su agenda para mejorar la atención de salud de los pobres. Se centra en la atención a los pobres y, particularmente, en el subprograma de atención primaria de la salud del MINSA, más que en reformas de todo el sector destinadas a una mayor eficacia. Se optó por esta concentración porque reducir la brecha entre el estado de salud de los pobres y de los otros niveles socioeconómicos es una prioridad declarada tanto del gobierno como del Banco. Al mismo tiempo, el entorno político y económico está cambiando de manera tal que podría poner en riesgo los adelantos logrados en la prestación de servicios a los pobres. La amenaza del terrorismo, que fue un incentivo importante para la creación de programas focalizados, ha disminuido. En el ámbito económico, los altos índices de crecimiento y la relativa abundancia fiscal que facilitaron la introducción de los programas focalizados se han visto afectados por las repercusiones de la crisis asiática.

Un tema central que resulta de este informe y aparece reflejado en sus conclusiones y recomendaciones es que sería de gran beneficio, en este nuevo entorno y ante los desafíos delineados anteriormente, mantener y profundizar las reformas destinadas a mejorar los servicios de salud para los pobres. Para que esto suceda, se tendrán que resolver problemas en la prestación, financiamiento, administración y dotación de personal de los servicios de salud. Estos problemas se sintetizan en este resumen ejecutivo y se describen en mayor detalle en los capítulos siguientes.

Reformas en la prestación de servicios de salud

Encuestas de hogares realizadas en 1997 demuestran que el MINSA gasta una cantidad similar *per cápita* en familias de bajos y de altos ingresos. Es decir que el gasto del MINSA es *neutral* en relación al ingreso, en lugar de ser *progresivo* concentrandose en los pobres. También señalan que los pobres reciben una mayor proporción del gasto en CPAPS que en hospitales. Está distribución del gasto se da a pesar que el gobierno ha

---

[1] Los intentos fallidos consistieron en leyes ambiciosas que intentaron separar el financiamiento de la provisión de servicios y reducir el exceso de empleo en el MINSA. También fracasó un intento de abrir la opción que los trabajadores asalariados pudiesen optar por abandonar totalmente el IPSS transfiriendo su cotización obligatoria a asegurados privados.

[2] Ha habido también algunos avances importantes para aumentar la competencia frente al IPSS, tales como: (i) la posibilidad de optar por no incluir en el IPSS una parte de la cobertura de salud (asignando un cuarto del impuesto sobre la planilla de pagos originalmente destinado al IPSS a EPSs privadas); (ii) la anulación del monopolio del IPSS sobre el seguro de riesgo para los trabajadores; y (iii) el desarrollo de sistemas de información que permiten el pago a cada hospital del IPSS a partir de los servicios producidos por el hospital, contabilizando en forma transparente cualquier subsidio que adicionalmente se asigne a ese hospital para cubrir su exceso de gasto.

introducido en años recientes importantes innovaciones que han logrado incrementar la prestación de servicios del MINSA para los pobres mediante: (i) la asignación de mayores recursos económicos a la atención primaria de salud; (ii) la asignación de fondos según los niveles regionales de pobreza; y (iii) el aumento de la participación de la comunidad en la administración de servicios. Estas innovaciones se presentan a continuación, conjuntamente con una indicación de sus debilidades. Hasta la fecha no se ha hecho ningún intento de orientar a los hospitales públicos, que funcionan actualmente de manera semicomercial, hacia una mayor prestación de servicios a los pobres.

El incremento del gasto en la atención primaria se logró mediante la creación de programas nuevos que utilizaron recursos frescos del tesoro, sin reasignar fondos existentes y sin introducir reformas en los programas y servicios tradicionales. Simplificando una estructura compleja, los proveedores de servicios del MINSA se pueden dividir en tres categorías, cada una de las cuales recibe financiamiento gubernamental a través de canales diferentes: Hospitales Nacionales, financiados directamente por el fisco; Hospitales Regionales financiados por el fisco a través de los gobiernos regionales; y CPAPS, financiados parcialmente a través de los gobiernos regionales y cada vez más a través de los programas focalizados. El presupuesto total del gobierno para estos proveedores se duplicó en términos reales durante 1994-97. La mayor parte del aumento se asignó a los programas focalizados, que recibieron un presupuesto de unos US$150 millones en 1998, o alrededor del 30% del total. El uso de fondos nuevos para financiar los programas focalizados postergó la necesidad de enfrentar a los grupos organizados en los servicios tradicionales. Esto, que fue una ventaja al permitir la rápida introducción de programas focalizados es hoy una fuente de vulnerabilidad. Bajo la situación actual, los programas nuevos probablemente serán los más afectados por las reducciones requeridas por una política fiscal más austera.

Un análisis de la distribución del presupuesto entre los diferentes departamentos del país señala que los programas focalizados asignan una alta proporción de sus recursos a los departamentos más pobres. En términos per cápita, las transferencias a los departamentos más pobres son cinco veces mayores que las que recibe Lima (el departamento más rico). Por el contrario, en términos per cápita, los presupuestos regionales se muestran altamente sezgados a favor de los departamentos más ricos. Si se suman los presupuestos regionales a los recursos de los programas focalizados, las transferencias del MINSA son proporcionales a la distribución de la población. Todavía existe amplia cabida para mejorar la asignación geográfica del 30% del presupuesto del MINSA destinado a los programas focalizados, mediante la mejora de los mapas de pobreza y mediante un mayor control para asegurar que los recursos se distribuyan eficazmente a las zonas más pobres. Las oportunidades más importantes de dirigir más recursos hacia los pobres no están al interior de los programas focalizados, sino en los servicios tradicionales y en particular en los hospitales. Es importante hacer esfuerzos por introducir medidas que permitan a los pobres beneficiarse más de los hospitales.

Con el fin de mejorar la eficacia en la atención primaria de la salud, se están desarrollando nueva formas de organización con la participación de la comunidad. La participación de la comunidad también podrían servir de catalizador para el desarrollo de grupos organizados que podrían ayudar a defender los programas nuevos contra reducciones presupuestarias. Estas reformas son necesarias, puesto que la productividad es baja y las actividades se instauran frecuentemente sin utilizar una evaluación diagnóstica local y a menudo se ven restringidas por reglamentos innecesariamente burocráticos. La baja productividad de los CPAPS es particularmente preocupante, ya que el promedio nacional es de 1 a 2 consultas clínicas al día por trabajador de salud. Es probable que los datos actuales subestimen los niveles de productividad al excluir o no contar la totalidad del trabajo preventivo y externo, pero incluso los cálculos conjeturales corregidos arrojan resultados muy bajos. Los CLAS son centros y puestos de salud administrados por la comunidad que implementan Programas de Salud Locales con financiamiento del Gobierno. Los indicadores disponibles sugieren que los CLAS, que administran actualmente 10% de las clínicas del MINSA, han dado buenos resultados en el aumento de la eficacia de la prestación de la atención primaria de salud. Estos buenos resultados se han logrado pese a la creciente oposición de las burocracias de los gobiernos regionales, que resienten la pérdida de control directo sobre los CPAPS y no proporcionan el apoyo técnico requerido a los CLAS. El otorgamiento de más permisos para la expansión de los CLAS ha estado congelado desde 1997 (pero podría reabrirse en un futuro cercano).

Reformas en el financiamiento de los servicios de salud

Los programas focalizados han logrado expandir la cobertura geográfica de los servicios de salud, al hacerlos funcionar y mejorar su calidad en zonas remotas. No obstante, muchos de los pobres todavía no tienen acceso a la atención de la salud debido a sus costos directos e indirectos. La mayoría de los proveedores del MINSA tratan de aliviar los costos para los pobres mediante exoneraciones parciales o totales del pago por concepto de **servicios**. Este sistema de exoneraciones tiene tres puntos débiles. En primer lugar, no existe un fondo para subsidiar medicamentos y suministros a nivel del proveedor, pero éstos constituyen más del 80% del costo directo de la atención médica para los pobres. La mayor parte de los medicamentos y suministros médicos, financiados por el centro médico a través de los cargos a los usuarios, se venden al usuario a su costo total más un margen de utilidad. En segundo lugar, la generosidad local financia las exoneraciones para los pobres. Puesto que no existe un medio para subsidiar específicamente a los pobres, cada centro financia los costos de ésta atención con sus propios recursos y toma voluntariamente la decisión de asignar tales recursos a la prestación de servicios a los pobres. Las necesidades son mayores en algunas zonas que en otras y no existen mecanismos que compensen esta disparidad. Por último, no existe ningún criterio ni metodología estándar para identificar a los pobres. Cada centro desarrolla su propio sistema y la mayor parte del tiempo lo aplica de manera irregular.

El gobierno ha empezado a afrontar el problema del costo para los pobres mediante la introducción de esquemas diseñados con el fin de proporcionar acceso a servicios cruciales para grupos seleccionados. El *Seguro Escolar* se creó en 1997 para cubrir servicios de salud y medicamentos para todos los alumnos de colegios públicos entre los 3 y los 17 años de edad (alrededor de 6 millones). El gobierno ha decidido crear un *Seguro Materno Infantil* (SMI), que cubriría servicios básicos para madres y niños menores de 3 años de edad, nutriendose de una creciente experiencia internacional que por ejemplo en Bolivia aumentó la cobertura institucional de partos en un tercio en sólo 18 meses. Ambos esquemas eliminan los pagos por los usuarios en el lugar de uso del servicio y cubren los medicamentos y otros insumos recetados. El Seguro Escolar es gratuito para los beneficiarios. El gobierno está estudiando la posibilidad de ofrecer el SMI, requiriendo el pago de una pequeña prima de seguro subsidiada (posiblemente gratuita en las regiones más pobres). Se piensa introducir el SMI como un esquema aparte; una vez consolidado, se establecería un solo esquema de seguros públicos que incorporaría el Seguro Escolar y posiblemente permitiría la opción de utilizar proveedores privados –en un primer momento ambos seguros están limitados a proveedores públicos.

Pese a los resultados positivos del Seguro Escolar, que cubrió 4 millones de atenciones durante 1998 y puede haber mejorado considerablemente la cobertura de escolares, y pese a los resultados prometedores de un pequeño experimento piloto con el SMI, el gobierno se muestra vacilante en crear y expandir el SMI. Las autoridades económicas están preocupadas por el costo. Algunos proveedores de salud vacilan como consecuencia de los problemas logísticos que se han presentado en la aplicación práctica del Seguro Escolar. Urge afrontar estos problemas para evitar que se creen cuellos de botella en el servicio y se desacredite un esquema prometedor. En el caso del Seguro Escolar, los reembolsos son lentos y los centros de salud se han visto forzados a cubrir muchos gastos con sus propios ingresos, ya que los reembolsos sólo cubren el costo de los medicamentos, mientras que los pagos directos por los pacientes cubren otros costos, incluyendo beneficios para el personal (tales como canastas de víveres).

Administración de programas dirigidos hacia los pobres

Existen ineficiencias en la administración de los programas claves del MINSA, lo que restringe su capacidad de establecer prioridades y prestar servicios de salud a los pobres. Muchos de estos problemas surgen de la fragmentación de los programas clave y de sistemas de información deficientes. El problema de fragmentación y duplicación es particularmente agudo en el control de programas de salud materno infantil, nutrición y salud ambiental. Ninguno de estos programas cuenta con una estructura directiva clara. En teoría, la política y planificación de las actividades materno infantiles es una de las muchas responsabilidades de la Dirección General de Salud de las Personas (DGSP). Dentro de la DGSP, esta responsabilidad está dividida en 8 programas nacionales. Dos proyectos grandes y muchos pequeños financiados externamente también financian éstas actividades. Cada uno de estos proyectos y programas lleva a cabo su propia planificación, desarrolla sus propios protocolos y planifica y financia sus propios programas de capacitación. En el caso de la salud ambiental, existen superposiciones y a menudo duplicaciones del control de calidad de alimentos y el control de la transmisión vectorial. En el área de la nutrición, se presentan superposiciones en las funciones desempeñadas por la DGSP, el INS y muchas otras instituciones públicas y privadas del sector fuera del MINSA. Un sistema presupuestario fragmentado sostiene esta duplicación.

La información sobre los gastos y sobre la producción de servicios de salud en el Perú es muy débil y los intentos de corregirla sufren de falta de continuidad y de consistencia. Pocos países en vías de desarrollo cuentan con un buen nivel de calidad en la información sobre el sector de salud, pero la mayoría tiene al menos información sobre el sector público. En el Perú no existe información consolidada sobre flujos financieros del sector público de salud, pues MINSA sólo conoce los gastos del departamento de Lima y ninguna agencia consolida los datos de otras regiones. Tampoco se conocen los datos sobre ingresos propios de los hospitales.[3] Las estadísticas de producción de los servicios han dejado de publicarse y de analizarse desde hace varios años. Los cálculos de consultas ambulatorias del MINSA para 1995 (las más recientes disponibles al momento de preparar este informe) fluctúan entre 15 millones (estadísticas oficiales) y 27 millones (cálculos a partir de encuestas de hogares). No existe una fuente de información oficial sobre consultas o internamientos en hospitales. Cada programa produce sus propios datos y se efectúan pocos intentos serios de consolidarlos de alguna manera que permita conocer y monitorear las actividades en conjunto (por ejemplo las actividades de control de la transmisión vectorial, las actividades de nutrición, hasta la producción en laboratorios, se miden por los diferentes programas de formas que no se pueden sumar ni comparar). Ocurren problemas similares con la medición de suministros, incluso partidas costosas como personal, capacitación o el abastecimiento de equipo, puesto que cada programa o fuente de financiamiento lleva sus propios registros y no existe una oficina de recursos humanos ni de infraestructura en el MINSA que consolide dicha información.

Recursos humanos para la atención de salud

Muchas de las ineficacias y disparidades en el sistema de salud tienen su origen en problemas de recursos humanos. De particular importancia para la prestación de servicios a los pobres son factores tales como distribución geográfica, mezcla de habilidades y calidad de los recursos humanos. La distribución geográfica ha mejorado notablemente en las últimas dos décadas, ya que el crecimiento en la población y los ingresos de las ciudades pequeñas ha propiciado que más médicos se establezcan en ellas. Más recientemente, los programas focalizados han colocado a más de 10,000 trabajadores de salud en zonas menos favorecidas. Estos programas ofrecen grandes incentivos económicos, pero el personal no recibe beneficios ni seguridad laboral. Pese a los incentivos económicos y a la sobre oferta temporal de los trabajadores de salud, la rotación de personal en las zonas remotas es sumamente elevado porque los sueldos más altos no compensan por el efecto combinado de la atracción de carreras profesionales vinculadas a la especialización médica y el ejercicio privado de la profesión que ofrecen las ciudades, y la carga de vivir en un entorno cultural radicalmente diferente. Esto se ve exacerbado por la ausencia de expectativas de una carrera de largo plazo en las zonas remotas, pues los contratos son breves. En vista de este dilema, los especialistas están buscando soluciones alternativas al problema de la atención de la salud de las comunidades rurales. Una opción que se viene estudiando implicaría un cambio en la combinación de habilidades de los trabajadores de salud locales, complementado por vínculos más fuertes con el resto de la red de salud. Los trabajadores locales asumirían más responsabilidades sobre el aspecto de salud pública, con un énfasis menor en los aspectos clínicos. Se necesitaría fortalecer las estructuras administrativas de los trabajadores locales, así como los sistemas de

---

[3] Hay en curso un intento de crear un sistema de cuentas nacionales de salud buscando superar los problemas de medición de intentos anteriores.

comunicaciones y de referencia y, en algunas zonas, se introduciría el uso de médicos móviles y "tecnología de telesalud".

El problema con la combinación de habilidades es que la formación médica no concuerda con el desplazamiento de las prioridades nacionales hacia la salud primaria y preventiva ni con el correspondiente desplazamiento hacia modelos de prestación de salud en el ámbito comunitario y rural. El desfase educativo se debe en parte a la atención relativa prestada a diferentes patologías médicas y en parte a la ausencia de conocimientos y habilidades de orden no médico relacionados con la salud pública y el trabajo comunitario. Asimismo, la formación de profesionales médicos no se ha mantenido al día con la rápidamente creciente importancia de los sistemas, el trabajo en equipo y la información en la prestación de servicios de salud y, por lo tanto, con la necesidad de desarrollar habilidades administrativas y directivas. El sistema educativo está empezando a responder a estos desfases, pero se necesitará de mayor esfuerzo y se necesita también dar señales claras a los jóvenes egresados y los estudiantes sobre las nuevas prioridades.

El consenso entre los funcionarios del MINSA y los profesionales médicos más eminentes es que la calidad de la educación médica se ha deteriorado. Mayormente, esto es un producto de la reciente creación a gran escala y poco reglamentada de facultades de medicina nuevas y el aumento en el número de institutos de enseñanza para técnicos de salud. Las universidades deben obtener licencias, pero en los últimos años los permisos de operación se han otorgado profusamente y, una vez en operación, las universidades no necesitan aprobaciones gubernamentales ni profesionales para otorgar títulos profesionales en medicina. Las licencias de centros educativos no universitarios no requieren aprobación ni certificación profesional.

Reformas propuestas

Las principales conclusiones de este informe son que las reformas introducidas por el MINSA para la prestación de servicios de atención primaria han rendido fruto y deben mantenerse, expandirse y profundizarse. Con ese fin, el informe principal presenta una serie de recomendaciones detalladas, que pueden agruparse bajo cinco encabezamientos claramente definidos de iniciativas de reforma: i) centrar más la atención en las necesidades de salud de los pobres al asignar fondos públicos; ii) reforzar la focalización entre los proveedores de salud del MINSA (mejor focalización de los programas y del gasto regional, mayor acceso por los pobres a servicios de hospitalización, mejor y mayor participación de la comunidad); iii) crear mecanismos de seguro médico nuevos para financiar la atención de la salud de los pobres; iv) mejorar los sistemas de información y gestión necesarios para ejecutar eficientemente y sin duplicación los programas de MINSA para los pobres; y v) afinar los requisitos de habilidades y los incentivos de los recursos humanos a fin de mejorar la ejecución de los programas orientados hacia los pobres.

Descripción del informe principal

Centrándose en los desafíos detallados anteriormente, este informe tiene la siguiente estructura. El Capítulo 2 reseña brevemente el sector de salud, con el fin de colocar al

MINSA y a las reformas recientes en una perspectiva más general (flujos financieros, el crecimiento de desembolsos para la salud y el acceso a los servicios, y un análisis de los subsectores beneficiados a partir de encuestas de hogar). El Capítulo 3 describe el progreso en los indicadores del estado de salud, así como un análisis de las diferencias entre los niveles y las necesidades de salud de los pobres y del resto de la población. El Capítulo 4 describe al MINSA en mayor detalle y analiza las reformas clave en la prestación de salud, tales como: el mayor énfasis en la atención primaria, el uso de la orientación a grupos específicos y los incentivos nuevos para mejorar la atención de grupos pobres, la gestión y la participación comunitaria. También plantea dos problemas fundamentales en los hospitales públicos. El Capítulo 5 analiza los obstáculos de costo y presenta dos esquemas actualmente en desarrollo para superar estos obstáculos: el Seguro Escolar y el Seguro Materno Infantil. El Capítulo 6 examina las deficiencias en la administración de los programas orientados hacia los pobres, con énfasis en la fragmentación y la ausencia de información. El Capítulo 7 analiza los aspectos relacionados con los trabajadores de salud. Primero analiza las tendencias principales en los mercados laborales para estos trabajadores y luego profundiza en temas de disparidad geográfica, calidad de la formación y la discordancia entre la mezcla de habilidades y las necesidades. En el Capítulo 8 se presentan las conclusiones y recomendaciones principales.

1.   EXECUTIVE SUMMARY AND INTRODUCTION

The Peruvian health sector has recovered rapidly after collapsing in the late 1980s and early 1990s as a result of hyperinflation and terrorism.   Total public and private spending on health rose by over 50% in real terms in the three years after 1994.   The supply of health services increased sharply, especially in primary care: the number of primary care clinics increased by two-thirds and their hours of operation were extended.   The employment of health professionals rose by 55%, mostly for primary care positions.   The demand for services also increased.   Nationwide, the use of services grew by over 55% in only three years.   In rural areas growth was almost 90%. Health outcomes have also improved rapidly in recent years. Infant mortality and child malnutrition, for instance, fell by almost a third during the first half of the decade and are likely to have continued to improve since. Despite these improvements in both inputs and outcomes, policy-makers face three key challenges and concerns.

First, how to *continue to reduce the large gap between the health status of the poor and that of the non-poor*. Peru is still an outlier in Latin America, exhibiting a very high IMR for a country with its level of income.   The high rates of infant mortality are concentrated among the poor.   Indicators for the higher income groups are close to the average for Latin America.   The poor, who are split between rural and urban areas, are made especially vulnerable to poor health by a combination of low levels of education, poor environmental conditions, and scant access to health services.   The poor suffer to a greater extent than the rest of the population from communicable diseases, many of which are exacerbated by environmental problems such as poor sanitation or vector infestation.   While their access to primary services for children over one month old has greatly improved in recent years, the poor continue to suffer from lack of access to services for mothers and young infants, who require primary and hospital-based services.

Second, how to *increase the resources assigned to provide care for the poor*. Peru continues to allocate fewer resources to health than most of its neighbors. The proportion of GDP assigned to health, –4.1% in 1997– is about two thirds of the Latin American average. The ratio of physicians to the population, –10 per 10,000– is only 70% of the Latin American average. There is also great inequality in the consumption of health goods and services.   Per capita consumption of health goods and services is approximately 4.5 times higher among the richest 20% of the population than among the poorest 20%. Whereas much of that difference is to be explained by greater amounts of private expenditure on health care by the rich, it is only partially offset by the Ministry of Health (MINSA), which in theory should be serving the poor, but in practice directs similar amounts to both the poor and the non-poor.

Third, how to *increase the efficiency in the use of these resources*.   Total health expenditures are around US$2.7 billion per year divided in equal parts between the private and public sectors (see Box 1-1). Approximately half of the public expenditures are channeled by MINSA, which assigns about a fifth of that to primary health care. There are very large inefficiencies in the system, reflected in the coexistence of extensive underutilized capacity in all sub-sectors with unmet needs and pent-up demand for some services. There are, above all, widely recognized inefficiencies due to fragmentation, lack of competition, and lack of separation between financing and provision. There are also significant inefficiencies in Primary Health Clinics (PHC), reflected in low productivity and insufficient adaptation to local needs.

Box 1-1

The Structure of the Health Sector

Peru's health system is a complex amalgam of several public programs and a private sector, each of which tends to go its own way, with little coordination or competition between program providers, in either financing or delivery of services. The main public programs are: the Ministry of Health (MINSA), financed by tax revenues and co-payments by users and providing services theoretically directed to the poor; and the Social Security Institute (formerly IPSS, currently ESSALUD), financed by a 9% payroll tax and theoretically covering all the health care needs of its formal-sector contributors. The private sector is financed almost entirely by out-of-pocket expenditures by households, as private insurance coverage is very small and the public programs (with very few exceptions) do not purchase services from private providers.

Household surveys show that MINSA plays a major role in the provision of clinical services, providing two-thirds of inpatient services and 44% of outpatient consultations. The private sector is also very important as a provider of outpatient services, in rural as well as urban areas and for the poor as well. IPSS, which accounts for 25% of national expenditure in health, provides 18% of outpatient services and 23% of inpatient services, all concentrated in the main cities and serving exclusively the non-poor.

A benefit incidence analysis was performed to understand the role of the different subsectors in serving the poor. Consumption of health care combines a private element with benefits channeled by MINSA and IPSS. Most of the inequality in health care consumption results from the assignment of greater amounts of private expenditure to health care by the rich than by the poor. This is reinforced by IPSS, which serves only formal sector employees and their families, who are concentrated in the higher echelons of the income distribution. MINSA expenditures reduce the overall inequality, but are not large enough or sufficiently well targeted among the poor to significantly equalize expenditures. The importance of MINSA is largest for the bottom 20%, who obtain 70% of their health benefits from this source compared to 20% for the richest quintile.

Several reforms have been tried during the years of recuperation of the sector. Some were successful, others failed. There were several failed attempts to pass legislation to introduce widespread reform in the sector to overcome the considerable inefficiencies created by the fragmentation, lack of competition and lack of separation between financing and provision that characterize the sector.[4] The most successful innovation consisted of building large

---

[4] The failed attempts included draft legislation to separate financing and provision and reduce excess employment in MINSA. There was also a failed attempt to allow formal sector workers to transfer their compulsory payroll contribution from IPSS to private insurers. While the attempts of "big bang" reform failed, important progress was achieved in introducing reforms to increase competition to IPSS, including: (i) the possibility of opting-out of IPSS for part of health coverage (assigning a fourth of the payroll tax originally earmarked for IPSS to private "health promoters"); (ii) the elimination of IPSS's monopoly over occupational risk insurance; (iii) the creation of insurance policies in IPSS for independent workers; and (iv) the development of information systems that allow for payment of each IPSS hospital based on services produced, and make explicit any additional subsidy paid to the hospital.

targeted programs to support primary care by allocating health workers based on regional priorities set by a poverty map, and by assigning funds for nutrition and to combat the diseases of the poor. In some areas the targeted programs have successfully piloted community participation.

This report is produced as an input to be used by the Government to continue to develop its agenda to improve health care for the poor. Its focus is on poverty, and particularly on ways to improve MINSA's primary health subprogram, rather than on sector-wide reforms to increase efficiency. This focus was chosen because reducing the gap in health status between the poor and the non-poor is a stated priority for both the Government and the Bank. The emphasis on incremental change, instead of widespread reform, was chosen because recent history suggests that the conditions are not ready for widespread reform but that much can be achieved with incremental changes, and these could become part of a broader reform in the medium term. At the same time, both the political and economic contexts are changing in a way that could jeopardize the progress achieved in providing services to the poor. The threat of terrorism, which was a major incentive for the creation of some targeted programs, has receded. The high rates of growth and relative fiscal abundance that facilitated the introduction of the targeted programs have been affected by the reverberations of the Asian crisis.

A leitmotif that emerges from this report and is reflected in its conclusions and recommendations is that much can be gained, in this new context and in response to the challenges outlined above, by sustaining and deepening the reforms directed toward improving health care for the poor. For that to happen, key outstanding issues in providing, financing, managing, and manning health services have to be resolved. These key issues are summarized here and described in more detail in the following chapters.

REFORMS IN HEALTH PROVISION

Household surveys for 1997 show that MINSA expenditures *per capita* benefit households of higher and lower incomes to a similar degree, instead of concentrating on the poor. They also show that the poor receive a larger proportion of the expenditure in Primary Health Clinics (PHC) than they do from hospital services. This pattern in the distribution of expenditures exists despite the introduction of successful innovations to increase the focus of MINSA service provision on the poor by: (i) increasing funding for primary health care; (ii) targeting funds according to regional poverty levels; and (iii) increasing community participation in running the services. These innovations are discussed below, with a brief indication of their remaining weaknesses. To date there have been no attempts to direct the public hospitals, which at present function in a semi-commercial way, to provide more services to the poor.

The increased funding for primary care was achieved by the creation of new programs using fresh funds and involving no reorientation of existing funds. MINSA service providers can be divided into three categories, each of which receives government financing through different channels: National Hospitals, funded directly by the treasury; Regional Hospitals funded by the treasury through regional governments; and PHC, funded partially through the regional governments and increasingly through the targeted programs created after 1994. The overall government budget for these providers doubled in real terms during 1994-97. Most of the increase was assigned to the newly created targeted programs, which received a budget of around US$150 million in 1998. The use of fresh cash to fund the targeted programs postponed any conflict with the powerful organized groups in the traditional services. Today the new programs are likely to take the larger cuts required by a tight fiscal stance.

An analysis of the distribution of the budget to the different Departments in the country shows that the targeted programs assign a large proportion of their resources to the poorest departments. In per capita terms, transfers to the poorest departments are five times larger than for Lima (the richest department). By contrast, in per capita terms the regional budgets are highly skewed in favor of the richer departments. Aggregating the regional budgets and the targeted programs, MINSA transfers are proportional to the distribution of the population. There is still ample room for improving the geographical targeting of the 20% of the MINSA budget which is assigned to the targeted programs, by improving the technical tools used to target and by strengthening controls to ensure that resources are effectively deployed to the poorer areas. To improve targeting of the overall MINSA budget would require politically more challenging changes, involving a reassignment of the budget directed to the hospitals.

New forms of organization, involving community participation, are being developed in an effort to increase effectiveness in primary health care. The reforms may also catalyze the development of organized groups that could help defend the new programs from budgetary cuts. These reforms are necessary, as productivity is low, activities are often implemented without use of a local diagnostic assessment, and they are often bound by unnecessarily bureaucratic rules. The low productivity of PHC is particularly worrisome, with a national average of 1-2 clinical consultations per health worker per day. Existing data underestimates productivity levels by excluding or undercounting preventive and extramural work, but even corrected guesstimates remain in a very low range. The CLAS are committees of community members who administer public facilities to implement population-based local health plans, financed by the Government. Most existing indications suggest that the CLAS, which today operate 10% of MINSA clinics, are successful as a means of increasing the effectiveness of primary care delivery. This success has been achieved despite a growing opposition from the regional government bureaucracies, which resent the loss of direct control over the clinics and are not providing the required technical support to the CLAS. The granting of new permits for the expansion of CLAS has been frozen since 1997 (but may be reopened shortly)

REFORMS IN HEALTH FINANCING

The targeted programs have succeeded in expanding the geographical coverage of health services by making services available and by improving their quality in remote locations. However, many among the poor remain without access to health care because of its direct and indirect costs. Most MINSA facilities make an attempt to address the cost barriers for the poor by providing partial or total exemptions from payment for **services**. This system of exceptions has its shortcomings. First, there is no fund to subsidize drugs and inputs at the provider level, and these constitute over 80% of the direct cost of health care for the poor. Most drugs and medical inputs, which are financed by the establishment out of revenues from user charges, are charged to the user at full cost plus a mark-up. Second, exceptions for the poor have to be financed by local generosity. As there is no instrument to have subsidies "follow the poor", each establishment finances the lost revenues from its own resources and the decision to assign these resources to provide services for the poor is voluntary. Third, there are no standard criteria or methodology to identify the poor. Each establishment develops its own system and applies it erratically most of the time.

The Government is beginning to tackle the cost barrier by introducing schemes designed to provide universal access by selected groups to key services. The *Seguro Escolar* was created in 1997 to cover health services and drugs for all children aged 3-17 attending public schools (around 6 million). The Government has announced the creation of a *Seguro Materno Infantil* (SMI), which would cover a package of basic services for mothers and for children under 3 years of age, following in the footsteps of expanding international experience in this area (a successful experience in Bolivia increased institutional coverage of births by a third in only 18 months). Both schemes eliminate co-payments by patients at the point of use of the service and cover prescription drugs. The *Seguro Escolar* is free of charge to beneficiaries. The Government is considering a small subsidized insurance premium (possibly free of charge in the poorest regions) for the SMI, which it plans to introduce as a separate scheme. Once consolidated, it would establish a single public insurance scheme incorporating the *Seguro Escolar* and possibly allowing a private provider option.

Despite positive results from the *Seguro Escolar*, which covered 4 million consultations during its first year of implementation and may have significantly improved coverage of school children, and despite promising results from a small pilot for the SMI, the Government is hesitant about expanding the SMI. The Ministry of Finance is concerned about its cost. Some health providers are hesitant because of logistic problems encountered in the implementation of the *Seguro Escolar*. These problems need to be addressed urgently to avoid creating bottlenecks in service and discrediting a promising scheme. In the *Seguro Escolar*, reimbursements are slow, and facilities have been forced to cover many expenses from their own revenues as reimbursements cover only the cost of drugs whereas the co-payments by patients covered other costs, including benefits for the staff (such as food baskets).

MANAGEMENT OF PROGRAMS DIRECTED TO THE POOR

The ability of MINSA to successfully prioritize and deliver health services to the poor is reduced because of inefficiencies in the management of key programs. Many of these problems arise from fragmentation of key programs and from weak information systems. The problem of fragmentation and duplication is especially acute for interventions in programs for maternal and child health (MCH), nutrition, and environmental health. None of these programs has a clear leadership structure. In theory, MCH policy and planning is one of many responsibilities of the *Dirección General de Salud de las Personas* (DGSP).

Within DGSP, this responsibility is split into 8 national programs. Two large and many small externally financed projects also finance MCH activities. Each of these projects and programs does its own planning, develops its own protocols, and plans and finances its own training programs. In environmental health, there are overlaps and often duplications in food quality control and vector control. In nutrition, overlaps occur in functions performed by DGSP, INS and many other public and private sector institutions outside MINSA. This duplication is underpinned by a fragmented budget system.

The weakness of the information on health service production in Peru is striking and past attempts to correct this have lacked continuity and consistency. Few developing countries have good quality data for the health sector, but most have information for the public sector. In Peru there is no attempt to consolidate information about financial flows or production services for the public sector. No agency collects or monitors information about expenditures incurred by all MINSA providers, or by all MINSA programs, or even by all externally funded programs.[5] Production statistics are no longer collected and published regularly. Estimates for MINSA ambulatory consultations for 1995 (the most recent available) run from 15 million (official statistics) to 27 million (household survey estimates). There is no official source for inpatient consultations. Each program produces its own data and there are few serious attempts to consolidate it in a way that would allow monitoring of activities at an aggregate level (e.g. vector control activities, nutrition activities, even laboratory production are measured by different programs in ways that cannot be aggregated or compared). Similar problems exists with the measurement of inputs, even for high-cost items such as staff, training, or the provision of equipment, since each program or funding source maintains its own records and there is neither a human resources nor an infrastructure office in MINSA to effectively consolidate such information.

HUMAN RESOURCES FOR HEALTH CARE

Human resource issues are at the root of many inefficiencies and inequities in the health system. Especially important for the provision of services to the poor are issues of geographical distribution, skills mix, and human resource quality. Geographical distribution has improved noticeably during the last two decades as physicians have been attracted to small cities as their population and income grew. More recently, the targeted programs have placed over 10,000 health workers in less-favored locations. These programs provide large financial incentives but workers have no benefits and no security in the job. Despite the financial incentives and the existence of a temporary oversupply of health workers, turnover in remote locations is exceedingly high as the higher incomes do not overcome the combined effect of the pull of professional careers, tied to city-based medical specialization and private practice, and the burden of life in a radically different cultural environment. This is exacerbated by the lack of expectations of a long-term career. This conundrum is leading specialists to look for alternative solutions to the problem of serving rural communities. One option under discussion would involve a change in the skills-mix for local health workers complemented with stronger links to the rest of the

---

[5] There exists an ongoing effort to produce national health accounts attempting to overcome the technical weaknesses of previous efforts.

health network. Local workers would be more in charge of the public health aspect of the job with less emphasis on the clinical aspects. Management structures for the local workers, communications and reference systems would need to be strengthened, and in some areas the use of mobile physicians and "telehealth technology" would be introduced.

The skill-mix problem is that the content of medical training has not kept up with the shift in national priorities toward primary and preventive health, or with the corresponding shift to community and rural health delivery models. The educational gap is in part a matter of the relative attention given to different medical pathologies, and partly of non-medical knowledge and skills related to public health and to community work. At the same time the training of medical professionals has not kept up with the rapidly increasing importance of systems, teamwork and information in health delivery, and therefore, with the need for administrative and managerial skills. The educational system is beginning to respond to these gaps, but additional effort will be needed.

The consensus among MINSA officials and medical professional leaders is that standards in medical education have been falling. This is mostly associated with the recent large-scale and little regulated creation of new university faculties in medicine and the increase in the number of teaching institutes for non-physician medical workers. Universities must obtain licenses, but permissions to operate have been granted liberally in recent years and, once in operation, universities need no further governmental or professional approval to grant professional titles to physicians. The licensing of non-university teaching centers is not subject to professional approval or certification.

PROPOSED REFORMS

The main conclusions of this report are that the reforms introduced by MINSA in the provision of primary care services have been successful and should be sustained, expanded and deepened. To accomplish that, the main report concludes with a chapter that makes a number of detailed recommendations, which may be grouped under five distinct reform initiative headings: i) establishing a sharper focus on the health needs of the poor in the allocation of public funds; ii) reinforcing that focus on the poor among MINSA health providers (improved targeting, increased access by the poor to hospital services, enhanced community participation); iii) creating new insurance mechanisms to finance health care for the poor; iv) improving the information and management systems needed to run MINSA's programs for the poor efficiently and without duplication; and v) refining human resource skill requirements and incentives to better serve poverty-oriented programs.

OUTLINE OF THE MAIN REPORT

Focusing on the challenges outlined above, this report is structured as follows. Chapter 1 is a brief overview of the health sector designed to put MINSA and the recent reforms in a more general perspective (financial flows, the growth in health expenditures and in access to services, and an analysis of which subsectors benefit different income groups). Chapter 2 describes the progress in health outcomes, analyzing differences in health status and needs between the poor and the rest of the population. Chapter 3 describes MINSA in greater detail and analyzes the key reforms implemented in health provision including: the increased emphasis on primary care, the use of geographical targeting, and new initiatives to improve management and community participation. It also discusses key issues in public hospitals. Chapter 4 analyzes the cost barrier and discusses two schemes currently being developed to overcome this barrier: the *Seguro Escolar* and the *Seguro Materno Infantil*. Chapter 5 examines ongoing shortcomings in the management of the programs directed to the poor, emphasizing fragmentation and lack of information. Chapter 6 examines issues related to health workers. It first analyzes the main trends in the labor markets for these workers and then discusses issues of geographical inequality, quality of training and the mismatch between skills-mix and needs. Chapter 7 brings together the main conclusions and recommendations.

2. OVERVIEW OF HEALTH SECTOR FINANCING AND DELIVERY SYSTEMS

Peru's health sector is a complex system is a complex amalgam of the following sectors:

- the Ministry of Health (MINSA), which finances and delivers care, in theory directed to the poor;
- the Peruvian Institute of Social Security (previously known as IPSS, recently renamed as ESSALUD), which finances and delivers care to formal sector workers and their dependants;
- several smaller public programs, including one for each branch of the military and another for the police, each of which finance and deliver care;
- a large private sector in terms of both delivery and financing of care; and
- several NGOs which mostly support the delivery of services by MINSA.

What follows is, first, a description of health expenditures and inputs in the sector as a whole. A second section describes the health infrastructure and staff available, their growth rates in the 1992-1996 period, and how they are distributed among the different subsectors. The third section documents the weight of the different subsectors in the provision of services. Fourth, a benefit incidence analysis is presented, describing how public and private expenditures are divided among the different income groups.

OVERVIEW OF HEALTH EXPENDITURES AND SYSTEM RESOURCES

During 1988-1993, financing for health fell drastically as a result of the drop in personal income and the collapse of all public expenditures brought about by the hyperinflation of the late 1980s and the stabilization policies used to control it in the early 1990s. Total spending in health has rapidly recuperated, increasing from US$1.6 billion in 1994 to over US$2.7 billion in 1997. Adjusting for inflation, this represented an increase of over 50% in real soles in only three years. Despite very rapid growth of GDP during these years, health expenditures grew faster than GDP, indicating a relatively high income elasticity (estimated at 1.29).

Table 2-1

Main Sources of Finance for the Health Sector, 1997

	US$million	Percentage of total	Percentage of GDP
Households spending	1,316	49	2.0
Government (taxes and loans)	690	26	1.1
Employers contributions to health insurance	682	25	1.0
Total	2,688	100	4.1

Source: Budget data and ENNIV 1997.

Despite this rapid recuperation, health expenditures in Peru continue to be low by any standard. As a fraction of GDP, health expenditures were only 4.1% in 1997 (Table 2-1). Estimates of the average for Latin America range from 5.5%-7.3%.[6] Per capita

---

[6] The low estimate is by the World Bank for 1994, and the high estimate is by PAHO for 1995. Only 6 countries in LAC spend as little on health as Peru.

expenditures in health, at US$90 per capita in 1997, are also about half of the Latin American average. Table 2-2 compares health expenditures for several countries in 1994.

Table 2-2

International Comparison of Health Expenditures (circa 1994)

	Peru (1994)	Bolivia (1994)	Brazil (1994)	Colombia (1994)	Ecuador (1994)	Mexico (1995)	Nicaragua (1994)	Panama (1994)
Health to GDP ratio (%)	3.7	7.1	4.6	7.4	5.3	4.2	8.6	67
Per capita expenditures on health (US$)	80	54	163	143	78	182	37	199
Per capita expenditures on health $PPP)	156	194	264	477	259	311	174	457
Public share (%)	60	58	40	40	39	56	61	70

Notes: Conversions to US$ based on official exchange rates. Purchasing Power Parities (PPPs) are exchange rates used to convert local currency into US dollars taking into account price differences across countries.

Source: Health and Population Indicators. World Bank, 1999.

MINSA is financed mainly by tax revenues, but it also obtains funds from external loans and from user fees. IPSS is financed by a 9% payroll tax paid by employers of formal sector workers. The smaller public programs are entirely funded by tax revenues. As in other countries of similar income level, in Peru about half of the health financing is provided by households, mainly as out-of-pocket payments. Private insurance covers less than 1% of the population and is often used as a complement to IPSS.

Table 2-3

Health Expenditures by Sub-Sector, 1997

	Real Increase 1994 to 1997	Per Capita Spending (US$)
MINSA	35	28
IPSS	19	105
Private	10	54
Total	55	90

Notes: The real increase was estimated in 1994 soles
Source: ENNIV 1994 and 1997. MINSA. IPSS.

MINSA, IPSS and households have all increased their spending substantially after 1994 (Table 2-3). The largest increase was in households' out-of-pocket payments for health care which doubled in real terms during 1994-97.[7] MINSA increased its spending by a third in real terms over this brief period. IPSS had the smallest increase, but even that meant a substantial increase in real terms in only 3 years.

Table 2-4 provides information on the physical configuration of the service delivery system in terms of personnel and facilities. MINSA has an important share of the assets and the staff in the sector. It runs the majority of the Primary Health Clinics (PHC), and while it accounts for less than a third of hospitals, these include most of the large hospitals, giving MINSA over half of the beds. It also employs over half of the health care professionals in the country, including 39% of physicians, most nurses, midwifes and auxiliary nurses. IPSS, with a stronger emphasis on secondary and tertiary service, has a small proportion of primary clinics, but a significant share of hospital beds and

---

[7] There is agreement that growth in private consumption was very rapid in this period, there is some disagreement about the magnitude of this growth, some of the apparent growth may be due to improved measurement.

physicians. The private sector is very large. Over 200 small formal private clinics employ a third of the physicians. Many of the physicians in public service also provide private services in single practitioner offices and other informal arrangements (these are not included in Table 2-4).

HEALTH CARE ACCESS AND USE

The years since 1992 have seen a sharp increase in the supply of health services, especially in primary health clinics (Table 2-4). The number of clinics increased by almost two thirds between 1992-96. FONCODES (Peru's social investment fund) alone rehabilitated or built 1, 213 primary care establishments for use by MINSA between 1992 and 1997 at a cost of about $30 million. Other agencies also contributed to this expansion of infrastructure. Growth has been rapid both in MINSA (where the number of establishments grew by 51%), in IPSS, and in the military. Additionally, MINSA and IPSS have established policies that have lead many clinics to significantly increase their hours of operation.

Table 2-4
Infrastructure and Staff of Health Services by Subsector in 1996

	Total 1996	Percentage Increase 1992-1996	MINSA	IPSS	Military/ Police	Private[1]	Total
Infrastructure			(% distribution 1996)				
PHC Facilities	6,717	61	86	3	2	9	100
Hospitals	472	4	30	15	4	51	100
Hospital Beds	42,979	n.a.	67	14	6	13	100
Staff							
Doctors	24,708	50	41	18	7	34	100
Nurses	16,139	45	58	23	10	9	100
Midwifes	5,105	120	77	12	3	8	100
Dentists	2,622	89	53	13	13	21	100
Technical Staff	44,742	n.a.	66	13	11	10	100

1/ "Private" refers exclusively to the corporate clinics.
Sources: CISRESA 1992 and CISRESA 1996.
n.a: not available

Table 2-5
Availability of Health Inputs, 1997 (per 10,000 population)

	Peru	LAC[1]	Andes
Physicians	10.3	14.9	13
Nurses	6.7	7.4	4.4
Dentists	1.1	5	3.8
Hospital Beds (per 1,000)	1.8	2.6	1.5

1/ Latin American Countries
Source: PAHO, Basic Indicators, 1998.

The availability of health professionals has also increased rapidly. Recruitment in professions such as midwifes and auxiliary nurses, who are required by primary clinics, has been particularly rapid. Despite this expansion, the low level of financing assigned to health care continues to be reflected in a low availability of physicians (only 70% of the Latin American average) and of other health workers such as nurses and dentists (Table 2-5). While Peru also has a lower number of beds per inhabitant than the Latin American average, it has more beds than neighboring countries, and there is significant excess capacity (only 52% occupancy).

Many Latin American countries invested heavily in health infrastructure during the 1990s, attempting to regain ground lost during the crisis of the 1980s. Some countries, such as Bolivia and Honduras have witnessed large growth of infrastructure accompanied by a proportionately much smaller expansion in effective coverage (in Honduras infrastructure grew by 40% and production increased by only 24%). Peru has been much more successful in translating physical expansion into improved coverage and effective use. Coverage for immunization and other preventive services has improved markedly (see Chapter 3). The use of ambulatory services —number of consultations—increased by 59% during 1994-97 (Table 2-6).[8] Inpatient services grew by 10% during that period.

Table 2-6

Use of Health Care in 1997

	Ambulatory Consultations in 1997		
	Total (million)	Increase 94-97	Per capita
Total	63.5	59%	2.6
Lima	22.2	99%	3.2
Other Urban	23.8	34%	2.7
Rural	17.5	58%	2.0
Source: Cuanto SA, based on ENNIV 1994 and 1997.			

MINISTRY OF HEALTH (MINSA), PERUVIAN SOCIAL SECURITY INSTITUTE (IPSS) AND THE PRIVATE SECTOR AS PROVIDERS

MINSA has a very large role in the provision of most types of health services. It is in charge of providing most public health interventions including organizing the whole immunization program and all vector control activities and sharing with municipalities responsibility for controlling the quality of water and food. MINSA also has a large role in the provision of clinical services, providing two-thirds of inpatient services and 44% of outpatient services. IPSS is the second most important provider of inpatient services, but has a much smaller role for the provision of outpatient consultations. By contrast, the private sector provides over a third of outpatient consultations, but only a small fraction of inpatient services.

Table 2-7
Importance of Providers by Region and Income Level, 1997 (%)

	Ambulatory					Hospitalizations				
	MINSA	IPSS	Military/ Police	Private	Total	MINSA	IPSS	Military/ Police	Private	Total
Lima	36	20	4	40	100	53	26	8	13	100
Other Urban	40	25	2	33	100	67	26	0	7	100
Rural	60	5	1	34	100	81	12	0	7	100
Quintile 1 (poorest)	68	4	1	28	100	85	0	0	16	100
Quintile 2	52	12	1	34	100	71	27	0	3	100
Quintile 3	53	15	1	32	100	65	26	0	9	100
Quintile 4	40	23	4	33	100	63	29	0	8	100
Quintile 5 (richest)	26	25	3	47	100	58	18	8	17	100
TOTAL	44	18	2	36	100	65	23	2	9	100

Source: ENNIV, 1997.

---

[8] The best definition of access would relate use to need. Unfortunately, LSMS surveys use only self-perceived illness as an approximation to "need." Self-perceived illness is influenced by expectations that tend to grow with income and education and has been shown to be poorly associated with burden of disease. Using self-perceived illness as an indicator would show that the largest increase in illness occurred in Lima and that Lima has the worst health status, followed by the Sierra (highlands) and, lastly, the Selva or Amazon jungle region (the opposite of what most analysts believe to be the case). By income level, the equally absurd pattern emerges that the richest quintile has the worst health status and the poorest quintile the best.

There exist some regional differences. MINSA is most important in rural areas of the Sierra (highlands) and the Amazon (Table 2-7). While it is less important in urban areas,

even there it is the single most important provider of health care. IPSS provides very few services to rural populations. The private sector is slightly more important in Lima than in the rest of the country, but it provides about a third of outpatient services in all regions (in remote rural areas this includes traditional practitioners).

There also exist differences by income group. MINSA is most important as a provider of services for the poor (Table 2-7). However, it is also significant as a provider for the non-poor. Lower income groups get most of their consultations from PHC centers, while users in the higher income groups use hospital outpatient facilities. MINSA's market share grew between 1994-97 for all kinds of services. This increase was especially large for the top 40% of households (D iagram 2-1).

IPSS beneficiaries are concentrated among the richer 40% of the population. Private providers are most important for the rich. However, they provide almost a third of outpatient consultations for the population as a whole.

D iagram 2-1

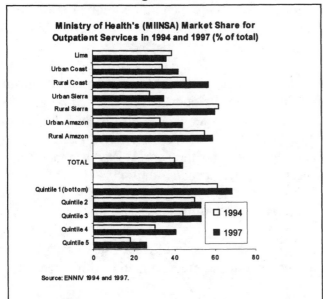

Source: ENNIV 1994 and 1997.

BENEFIT INCIDENCE OF HEALTH EXPENDITURES[9]

Per capita consumption of health goods and services is about 4.5 times higher in the top quintile than in the bottom quintile (Diagram 2-2). This difference, while very large, is less than the difference in total consumption (a ratio of 1:7.5). The consumption of health care combines a private element with benefits channeled by MINSA and IPSS. Most of the inequality in health care consumption results from the assignment of greater amounts of *private* expenditure to health care by the rich than by the poor (top to bottom quintile ratio of health expenditures of 1:10). This is a common pattern as health care is a good whose consumption normally rises with income or faster.

---

[9] Benefit incidence analysis combines the cost of providing public services with information on their use in order to generate distributions of the benefit of government spending. This has become an established approach since the path-breaking work by Meerman (1979) on Malasia and Selowsky (1979) on Colombia. The benefit incidence analysis presented in this study involved a three step methodology. First, estimates were obtained of the unit subsidy of: (i) consultations in PHC, (ii) ambulatory consultations in hospitals, and (iii) inpatient consultations in hospitals. These estimates were obtained based on 1997 budgets and 1997 ENNIV utilization data. Second, the unit subsidy was distributed to individuals who were identified from ENNIV as users of the service. Third, individuals were aggregated into five quintiles (each including a fifth of the population) based on the total per capita expenditures of the household.

Diagram 2-2

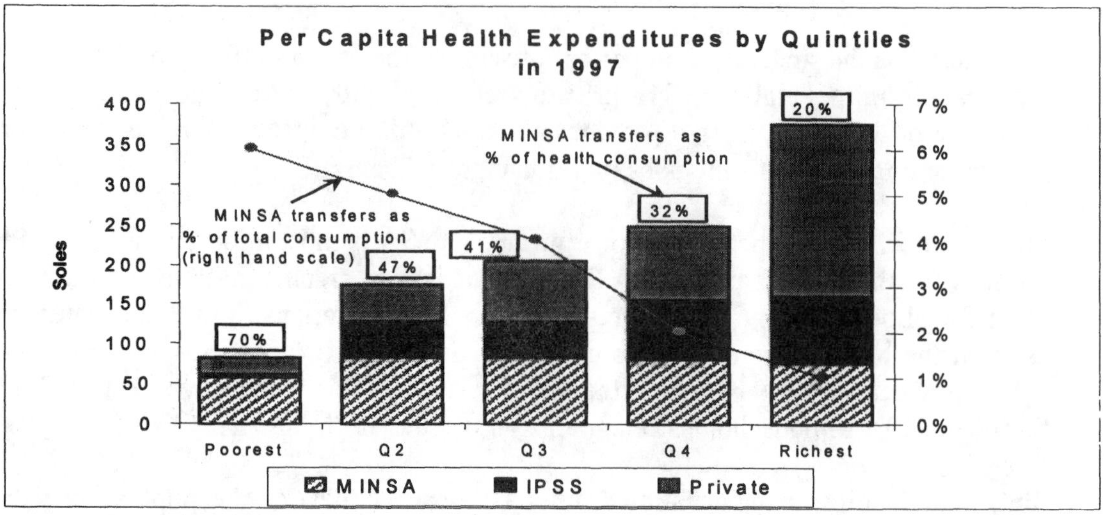

Per Capita Health Expenditures by Quintiles in 1997

Source: World Bank Estimates described in footnote 9.

The inequality in the consumption of health benefits is reinforced by IPSS, which serves mostly formal sector employees and their families and these are concentrated in the higher echelons of the income distribution.[10] MINSA expenditures reduce the overall inequality, but are not large enough or sufficiently well targeted among the poor to significantly equalize expenditures.

The distribution of MINSA expenditures is almost proportional to the population, in the sense of similar nominal amounts being directed to the poor and to the non-poor. The poorest 20% of the population receive a slightly lower per capita subsidy than the rest of the population. However, in proportion to their income this benefit is significantly higher for this group than it is for the rest of the population: for the poorest it adds about 5% to their total consumption; for the richest quintile, it adds only 1% to their total consumption. The importance of MINSA is largest for the bottom 20% who obtain 70% of their health benefits from this source compared to 20% for the richest quintile.

In this chapter the focus has been on financing and provision of health services. We now turn to a discussion of the progress made and ongoing shortcomings in health outcomes.

---

[10] Within the formal sector workers, IPSS may bring some progressivity. Indirect calculations based on ENNIV (which did not ask for information about social security contributions) suggest that the top quintile may be paying around 51% of IPSS revenues and is benefiting from 33% of expenditures. The bottom 60% may be contributing to 26% of the cost and receiving 38% of the benefits.

3. PROGRESS IN HEALTH OUTCOMES

Like other countries in the region, during the last 25 years, Peru has experienced a slowdown in population growth and a strong trend toward urbanization. There has also been improvement in the health status and life expectancy of much of the population. In this regard, recent years have seen important achievements in some areas combined with great deficiencies in others. This chapter describes the main achievements in health status and identifies shortcomings, with emphasis on the health needs of the poor.

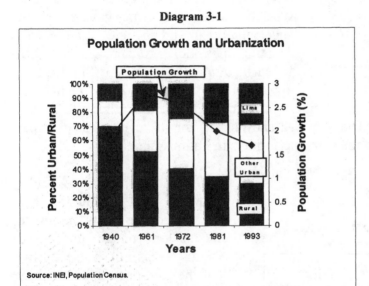

Diagram 3-1

Source: INEI, Population Census.

Population growth had slowed down to 1.9% per year in 1996, reducing the gap with other Latin American countries which grew on average by 1.5%. The mobility of the population has continuously increased, and the 1993 census revealed that almost a fourth of the population is migrant. The high rates of rural to urban migration that accompanied the drop in population growth have created a country where 70% of the population now lives in cities or on their periphery (Diagram 3-1). The share of the population living in the highlands has fallen, and that of the Coast and the Amazon continues to expand. A key feature of the country continues to be the primacy of Lima, which still accounts for over half of the urban growth and is ten times larger than the second largest city (Arequipa).

Table 3-1

Health Indicators, 1991-1996

Indicators	1991	1996	Difference (%)
Infant mortality rate (per 1000 live births)	60	43	- 28
Under -5 mortality rate (per 1000 live births)	80	59	- 26
Chronic malnutrition (% of children < 5 yrs)	37	26	- 30
Maternal mortality rate (per 100,000 live births)	298	265	- 11
Total fertility rate	4.0	3.5	- 13
Life expectancy in years	64	68	+ 6
Post-neonatal mortality (per 1000 live births)	29	19	- 35
Neonatal mortality (per 1000 live births)	29	24	- 17

Source: ENDES 1992 and 1997.

Child and infant mortality indicators improved by more than a fourth since 1990 (Table 3-1).[11] Much of the progress was attained by a significant increase in immunization coverage (especially measles) and the control of diarrheal disease in children.

---

[11] The most recent data available are from a survey undertaken in 1996. This survey collects data on health outcomes for 1991-1996. Hence it does not fully reflect the impact of the expansion in coverage described in Chapter 1.

Table 3-2
Coverage of National Programs , 1991-1996
(Percentage)

Indicator	1991	1996
Childhood programs		
All vaccinations (12-23 mo.)	58	63
Vaccinations (12-23 mo.):		
Polio (3 doses)	69.9	71.4
DPT (3 doses)	68.1	77.0
Measles	74.0	85.8
BCG	90.6	94.3
Diarrhea cases utilizing ORT (< 5 yr)	31.1	55.3
Exclusive breastfeeding (0-3 mo.)	40.5	61.7
Safe Motherhood Programs		
Tetanus toxoid-2 doses in pregnancy	20.1	51.3
Antenatal care	64	67
Skilled childbirth attendance	52	56
Modern contraceptives (% of couples)	33	41

Source: ENDES 1992 and 1997.

(Table 3-2). Diarrhea-related deaths have fallen noticeably following the strong hygienic practices and ORT (oral rehydration therapy) educational campaigns for the public and for health workers that were launched during and after the cholera epidemic. Considerable effort has gone in recent years into improving water and sanitation with investments that by 1997 had surpassed $100 million.[12] New vaccines have been added to the program (Hepatitis B and Haemophilus influenzae type B).[13] Malnutrition rates have decreased substantially in urban and rural areas. Stunting of children under age five has fallen in rural areas from 53% in 1991 to 40% in 1996, and from 26% to 16 % in urban areas.[14] Despite this important progress in child health, Peru continues to have a very high infant mortality rate. Diagram 3-2 shows that, for its level of income per capita, Peru continues to be one of the worst performers in Latin America.

Diagram 3-2

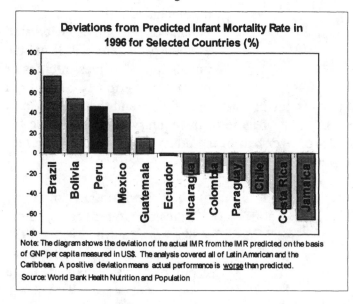

While the health of older infants and children has improved markedly, the health status of young infants and mothers has not. The progress of the past decade was mainly in post-neonatal mortality related to more prevention and better clinical management of infections; much less progress was achieved in perinatal or maternal mortality. The maternal mortality rate for 1992-96 of 265 deaths for 100,000 births is almost one and a half times higher than the LAC average and is 15 times the average for developed

---

[12] Less progress has been made with child mortality related to respiratory infections (ARI): symptoms of severe ARI continue not to be widely recognized by the population and help-seeking is frequently delayed; medication although free-of-charge is often not available in public clinics; frontline health workers are often insufficiently trained to handle cases and to refer them to higher level facilities, referral systems are ineffectual; and (despite the progress claimed by some official statistics) intra-hospital mortality for pneumonia continues to be significantly high. On the positive side, the incidence of pneumonia is expected to fall following the introduction of Hib vaccine in 1999.

[13] Official statistics claim that 96% of children received all their vaccines in 1996. Survey data suggest that these claims are exaggerated by around 30%, but confirm that there has been an improvement in coverage.

[14] ENDES 1991 and 1996. ENNIV, using a different methodology also found a substantial improvement in malnutrition between 1994 and 1997.

countries. The main causes of maternal death (hemorrhage 23%, mishandled abortion 22%, infections 18% and hypertension 17%) suggest that much of the problem lies in inadequate conditions at the time of birth both at home and in the hospital. Though case-fatality rates for home births are much higher than for hospital births, birth-fatality rates in hospitals are five times that of developed countries. Maternal mortality due to unreported illegal abortion is undoubtedly a larger problem than has been officially diagnosed, especially in urban areas. There has been a large push for family planning during 1997 and 1998. However, coverage remains low. The quality of Ante-natal Care (ANC) is unknown as its content is not well controlled. Even less progress has occurred in second level obstetric care. Coverage of births by skilled health workers remains at around one-half of the total; in rural areas professional birth attendance is only 22%. Perinatal mortality is related in large part to inadequate conditions in labor and delivery, but also to poor maternal obstetrical, medical, and nutritional antecedents that result in prematurity, low birth weight, or worse if needed interventions are not available. More prevention is needed in maternal health in addition to the current focus on improving obstetrical health service capacity.

The extremely low levels of use of health services by mothers are partly a reflection of ethnic and cultural barriers, combined with low levels of female education and cost barriers. However, they also reflect the low priority assigned to Safe Motherhood interventions.[15] Also, there has been no attempt to limit the direct and indirect cost to the patient of using obstetric services (although there is now a plan to create the new *Seguro Materno-Infantil* –see Chapter 4). In consequence, coverage of births by skilled personnel is still a problem even in urban areas. The cultural barrier in rural areas is heavily reinforced by staff that remain unprepared to deal with poor indigenous women, who especially object to unaccommodating birthing conditions and fear various other aspects of institutional care. There are serious weaknesses in safety and quality assurance (Box 3-1). These received a great deal of publicity in relation to complications arising from surgical sterilization operations carried out as part of the family planning program of 1998. Part of the problem was due to low quality of surgical care and part was due to the lack of capacity to communicate with mothers and especially indigenous mothers.[16]

---

15 A "National Plan of Action for the Reduction of Maternal and Perinatal Mortality 1998-2001" was recently launched with external support. It remains small and isolated from the main initiatives in the sector. This may be corrected in the near future by combining this effort with the creation of the Seguro Materno Infantil.

[16] A special commission set up to investigate the charges found that few of the cases reported were due to medical negligence. It recommended, in general, the need to provide additional training, require that only specially-trained personnel perform surgical procedures, and ensure that all women are properly informed as to possible complications and the need for follow-up visits. What should be stressed, rather than goals related to the number of new users of any given method, is the number of protected couples (users move in and out of contraceptive use very fast). Another problem is the quality of care, in providing for client choice of method and full information on method use and potential side effects.

Box 3-1

Utilization of Obstetrical Services in Rural Peru

Utilization of maternal health services depends on: i) women's and husbands' *perceptions* of need, accessibility, and quality of care; ii) accessibility; and iii) quality of care. The following are the results of a study* on reproductive health care based on 917 women interviewed in 12 rural villages of Huancavelica, the Department with the highest maternal and infant mortality in Peru.

Prenatal care

- A significant increase in prenatal care occurred between 1992 (12%) and 1997 (80%) due to: i) increased availability, and ii) need to complete an eligibility requirement to receive supplementary foods or other benefits. Afterwards, many did not return for further visits.
- Principal reasons given by women for not using prenatal care were: fear or distrust of health personnel, it was considered unnecessary, and the service did not exist (ceased to be a major reason in 1995-1997).
- Women did not identify pregnancy and childbirth as events requiring preventive health services. As long as a pregnant women could continue domestic, agricultural, and animal-raising activities, she considered herself healthy. People were not accustomed to using the health facility, and much depended on the personal relationship between the health worker and the individual woman. Health services were associated with curative care, although they were not seen as well prepared to carry out this role.
- Only 64% of 12 facilities had minimum equipment for provision of prenatal care.

Delivery assistance

- Only 2% of births were institutionally attended. Eight percent were attended by health personnel.
- The major reason cited for not delivering in a health facility was that it was not considered necessary, despite the fact that well over half the women reported complications with their last delivery (excessive bleeding, > 12 hours of labor, fever, convulsions, or other). Secondly, women cited reasons of fear or distrust of health personnel: including fear of male providers, fear of being chastised or insulted, and fear of intervention (e.g. c-section). Institutional deliveries were associated with a cold environment, strange persons, or unfamiliar activities that could provoke complications of 'cold' and '*susto*' (fear).
- The husband usually helped with delivery and played a major role in health care decisions. Use of traditional midwives was rare.

Perceptions of health post personnel

- Health post personnel recognized that communities have strong belief systems regarding certain health issues, and felt incapable of dealing with them.
- They complained of a shortage of equipment and supplies, but also recognized their limited technical capacity to deal with many health problems, citing a need for more professional personnel.
- Most complained of being over-worked, often being the only staff to attend patients in clinic, visit annex communities for program activities, as well as fill out many reporting forms.
- Many were contracted for 3-6 months before reassignment elsewhere, impeding development of personal relationships. Personnel assigned for longer periods had more positive experiences with the community.

---

*Source: L. Altobelli and F.R. León (1997) *Changing community perceptions of reproductive health services and reducing the unmet need for them in Peru's highland: I. A baseline study.* Final Report of INOPAL III Sub-Project. Lima: Population Council.

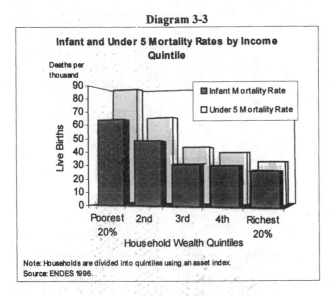

Diagram 3-3

The highest mortality rates are concentrated among the poor and in rural and peri-urban areas. Infant and child mortality levels for the richer 60% of the population are at levels comparable to the LAC average. The real problem in Peru is concentrated among the poorer 40% of the population, where almost 60% of child deaths occur (Diagram 3-3).[17] Poor households are handicapped by a combination of low education and worse environmental conditions. They also have less access to some key health services. Communicable diseases are considerably more common as a cause of death for the poor than for the non-poor. They account for almost half of deaths in the poorest quintile compared with about a fifth of deaths for the richest quintile. Non-communicable diseases are correspondingly less important for the poor (Diagram 3-4).

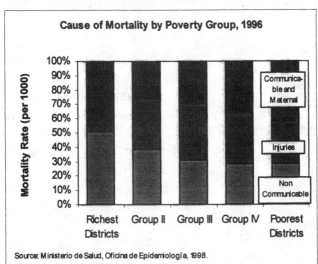

Diagram 3-4

Diagram 3-5 shows how access to key child health interventions, which are provided free of charge and with monitored target coverage, such as vaccinations and appropriately treated diarrhea, have expanded and are fairly homogeneous across income levels (ARI treatment excepted). By contrast, the poor continue not to have access to services provided on demand (and which are more complex in terms of equipment, supplies, technical capability, counseling needs, and continuing patient follow-up, such as safe obstetrical and postpartum interventions, which impact on maternal and perinatal mortality).

---

[17] The data used here were processed by Macro International Inc. under contract with the World Bank's thematic group on poverty and health. The estimates are from the 1996 *Encuesta de Demografía y Salud* (ENDES), a household survey undertaken as part of the multi-country Demographic and Health Survey (DHS) Program. The quintile divisions are based on an asset index created as a proxy for wealth and income.

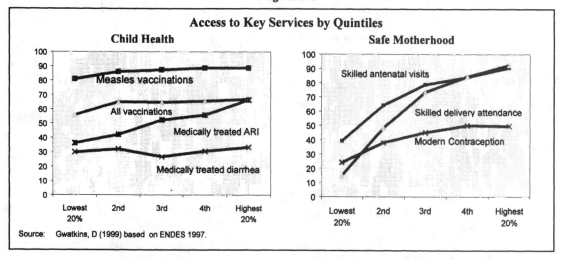

Diagram 3-5

Access to Key Services by Quintiles

Source: Gwatkins, D (1999) based on ENDES 1997.

Many of the poor live in rural areas and the vulnerability created by poverty and poor nutrition is accentuated by the problems of access to services and by the environmental challenges of rural areas. Rural infant and child mortality rates are twice as high as in urban areas (Table 3-3).[18] [19] As in the case with the poor, in rural and peri-urban areas, the main cause of death continues to be infectious diseases (including ARI, diarrheal diseases, and tuberculosis — frequently accompanied by some degree of malnutrition). The worse indicators are from areas that combine poor environmental conditions and low levels of education. Illiteracy among rural women is four times higher than among urban women.

Table 3-3

**Indicators of Maternal and Child Health:
Urban-Rural Comparison (circa 1994)**

Indicator	Urban	Rural	Relation Rural/Urban
Infant mortality (under 1 yr)	30	62	2.1
Child mortality rate (under 5 yrs)	40	86	2.1
Stunting (height for age < 5 yrs)	16	40	2.5
Birth rate (per 1000 inhabitants)	24.2	33.5	1.4
No prenatal care (%)	18.6	53.2	2.9
Non-professional birth attendance	19.4	78.5	4.0
Female illiteracy (%)	6	24	4.0
No indoor water connection (%)	28.3	74.5	2.6
No indoor toilet (%)	33.4	96.6	2.9
Crowding (5+ persons / bedroom)	13.9	27.8	2.0

Source: ENDES 1997.

A long-term view of trends suggests that the rural/urban demographic and educational differences are slowly being reduced. However, less progress is being achieved in reducing the nutritional and environmental risk factors in peri-urban and rural areas. While the rural/urban education gap will remain wide, today's enrollment rates of rural girls and the age structure of illiterate women

---

[18] Statements about peri-urban areas are based on interviews with specialists. Epidemiological studies break down their data into urban and rural, and present no results for peri-urban areas, which today may hold as much as a third of the population. This is a major weakness of these data.

[19] As explained above, the 1997 DHS reports on health status for 1991-1996, which does not fully reflect the benefit of the recent expansion.

imply that the levels of female illiteracy among fertile-age women will drop sharply for the next generation.[20] Also, the cultural gap is being reduced as rural groups, with greater access to education and mass media become better aware of national standards of social and cultural behavior. Despite some progress in expanding water and sanitation, a large part of the population remains under-served. Unsanitary conditions for food, waste and other forms of pollution are rapidly rising in peri-urban and rural areas and there is no concerted effort to confront this. In addition, rural and peri-urban populations are increasingly at risk from the reemergence of communicable diseases.

Over the last decade there has been a resurgence of communicable diseases once thought to be under control, accompanied by the appearance of new diseases. On the increase, or on their way to becoming chronic problems are: malaria of the *Falciparum* variety; the development of multi-drug resistance to tuberculosis; yellow fever; dengue; cholera; rabies; and the appearance of HIV/AIDS (see Box 3-2). Peru's diversity, in terms of its geography and climate and its social and cultural heterogeneity make the country particularly vulnerable to many of these diseases. This vulnerability has been accentuated in recent years by the convulsion created by terrorism, which led to the displacement of a significant fraction of the population, exposing it to new health risks and creating environmental changes in urban and rural areas. The economic crisis that accompanied the terrorist upheaval also contributed to the deterioration of public health programs. The vulnerability has also increased because of long-term structural change in the environment and in the economy, specifically by: ecological changes created by deforestation, agricultural development and irrigation; increased permanent and seasonal migration into the Amazon in search of new economic opportunities; increased contacts with the population of neighboring countries associated with the expansion of licit and illicit trade; misuse of antibiotics and other antimicrobial drugs; and cyclical changes in climate and weather (especially as regards the spike in vector-born and infectious diseases in 1998 related to the *El Niño* phenomena).

Box 3-2

Emerging and Re-emerging Diseases in Peru

Vector-transmitted diseases

- In 1998, 216 thousand cases of **malaria** were notified, with 37% of those being of the *Falciparum* variety, notorious for its lethality and resistance to drugs. The highest incidence of *Falciparum* is in Loreto in the Amazon region. Due to the El Niño phenomenon, Piura had a significant outbreak in 1998, but the overall number of cases in the country was similar to 1997. *Vivax* malaria is often ignored due to its lower virulence, but is easily as important as the other form due to its characteristic recurrence and impact on social and economic life of entire villages. Malaria has been developing as a major problem since the early 1990's.
- There have been several localized epidemic outbreaks caused by the **Dengue** virus since 1990; 1,311 cases were notified in 1997, diminishing to 986 cases in 1998. The risk of new epidemics, including of the hemorrhagic type, persists in the areas where home-infestation by the vector are common (mainly in the Amazon).

---

[20] Other features will bring disadvantages for rural areas. Part of the differential in rural/urban growth is a statistical artifact by which rural settlements grow beyond the 2,000 divide or cross over some other arbitrary line and become classified as urban. Those still classified as rural are likely to be more dispersed than before. This will make them harder to serve with water and sanitation, education, or health services.

- There have been over 10 outbreaks of **yellow fever** since 1991. While only 43 cases were notified in 1997, this increased to 165 cases (with 49 deaths) in 1998. The increase is related to migration towards endemic areas for the cultivation of coffee.
- **Bubonic plague** remains endemic in the departments of Piura and Cajamarca since 1903, with a cyclical behavior. In 1997, 37 cases were notified in Cajamarca, Lambayeque and La Libertad, while this was reduced to 21 cases in 1998.

Other Diseases

- In 1998, 3 cases of **measles** were confirmed by laboratory analysis to have occurred in Ancash (1), Lima (1), and Arequipa (1). Six cases had been reported in 1997.
- A total of 13 cases of **neonatal tetanus** were notified in 1998.
- **Cholera** is unusually persistent in Peru, despite great efforts to control it. Largely due to the El Niño phenomenon in 1998, as many as 42,083 cases were reported (with 389 deaths), in contrast to 1997 when only 3,284 cases were notified.
- **Rabies** is endemic in Peru. In 1998, there were 9 cases of rabies in humans, spread over 6 departments, down from 12 cases in 1997.
- **AIDS**: 428 cases were notified in 1997; most of them in Metropolitan Lima. Part of the increase is due to improved case identification and reporting. The speed of growth of HIV infection is thought to have been reduced in recent years.

The most recent complete data from the national **tuberculosis** program show 47,062 cases reported in 1997, with slightly fewer cases in 1998. Reported cases are concentrated in Lima and Callao. TB is soon to become a notifiable disease in the national epidemiologic surveillance system.

An additional point needs to be emphasized: large cities have a lower proportion of deaths occurring in childhood and a much greater proportion of chronic and degenerative diseases of old age. While the population over 65 years of age is only 5% of the total nationally, it is larger in metropolitan areas and is projected to double in those areas over the next twenty years which will place a heavy burden on government health services for high cost surgical and recuperative care. MINSA is currently lacking promotional health programs to prevent these diseases, some of which can be avoided by early adherence to healthier lifestyles (better eating habits, exercise, reduced stress, no smoking or alcohol, and others). Prevention and screening for cervical, breast, and prostate cancer (and treatment when required) is another important area to which MINSA needs to pay attention.

4. REFORMS IN HEALTH PROVISION

This chapter will review some of the key determinants that explain the distribution of benefits from MINSA services between the poor and the rest of the population and will discuss important reforms recently introduced by MINSA to improve the way it reaches the poor. The chapter begins by looking at the distribution of MINSA's expenditures among the population. It then proceeds to describe MINSA's structure, spending, and programs, particularly those designed to serve the poor. One of the key reforms in the provision of services has been the explicit introduction of targeting of direct investments to the poor. We then discuss the extent to which public expenditures are accurately and effectively targeted. A fourth section of this chapter analyzes issues of efficiency in the delivery of primary care, while a fifth section looks at new initiatives to improve management and community participation in primary health clinics: the CLAS and the health networks (*Redes*). An area that has been left largely untouched by reforms is the large hospital sector. The last section describes some of the future challenges in reforming public hospitals to increase their usefulness to serve the poor.

MINISTRY OF HEALTH AND THE DISTRIBUTION OF HEALTH BENEFITS

Diagram 4-1

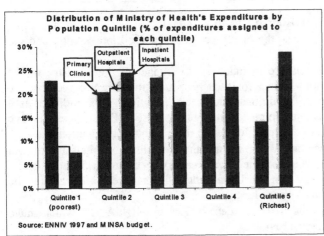
Source: ENNIV 1997 and MINSA budget.

In Chapter 1, we showed that MINSA expenditures are almost proportional to the population, instead of being targeted to the poor or biased in favor of the rich. Within MINSA there exist important differences as some of the MINSA programs are more pro-poor than others. MINSA primary health clinics have the most progressive distribution of services (Diagram 4-1). This is the only program where the fraction of expenditures assigned to the bottom 20% is higher than for the top 20%.

Ambulatory service in hospitals has an intermediate impact; while it does not reach the poorest quintile, it does benefit all the rest of the population in a similar fashion. Hospitalizations (inpatient services) also benefit the whole population, but, in contrast to the other services, these benefits are largest for the top quintile, while only 8% are assigned to the bottom quintile and some of these services are provided by primary health centers with beds, rather than by hospitals. This bias in favor of the rich is likely to be even larger than what is measured in Diagram 4-1 because the rich tend to use public hospitals only for high-cost services provided by the specialized hospitals, preferring private hospitals for simpler inpatient services such as birth delivery and basic surgery.[21]

MINISTRY OF HEALTH: STRUCTURE AND EVOLUTION OF EXPENDITURES

Peru is divided into political Regions responsible for the provision of most public services, including health care. MINSA's central office is only responsible for the financing and provision of services in the Lima Region which includes Metropolitan Lima (the city of Lima and the port of Callao) and the Department of Lima. The regional authorities are appointed to the Ministry of the Presidency (MINPRE) in consultation with MINSA. Their budgets, including the requirements for the regional health services, are included in the MINPRE budget. While MINSA in theory is responsible for policy and planning nationally, in practice it has little influence over activities financed through MINPRE.[22]

While the deconcentration of budgets to the regions had been expected to lead to an adaptation of expenditures to local needs, over the years the regional authorities have reinforced the traditional structure of the health sector they inherited. Most of their funding is assigned to the payment of staff in regional hospitals and in the regional administration. Negligible amounts are assigned by the regions to primary health clinics or to environmental health. The existing budget structure is described in Box 4-1.

Box 4-1

Structure of the Ministry of Health's Budget

- *MINSA Headquarters (HQ)*. Its budget finances the health providers in the Lima Region and the central administration.
- *MINSA Regions*. The regional health budgets are included in the budget of the Ministry of the Presidency (MINPRE) as part of the overall budget for each region. Funds are provided for the payroll and some fixed costs. Allocation of additional funds for discretionary expenditures is a decision of the Region. Payments to the regions are made directly from MEF. MINSA does not have any participation in the budget process. It is not even informed of regional budget execution.
- *The National Hospitals*. Each of these Hospitals (which include the specialized hospitals and the old and prestigious hospitals that used to belong to the *Beneficencia*) is budgeted independently. Although the budget entry is registered as part of the Lima budget, in practice the budget for the National Hospitals is managed independently by each hospital.
- *The Targeted programs*. These programs have independent offices in MINSA HQ which make transfers for specific activities carried out by the regions.

---

[21] Because of limitations in the data, the diagram is based on the single assumption that all hospital services have the same unit cost.

[22] A 1998 law (*Ley Marco de Descentralización*) eliminated this organization, which had been in place for a decade and was based on regions consisting of several Departments, making all public health services dependent on MINSA and centralizing all budget planning and monitoring in MINSA. This lasted for a few weeks, after which the previous system was reestablished by Congress (but with Regions consisting each of a single Department).

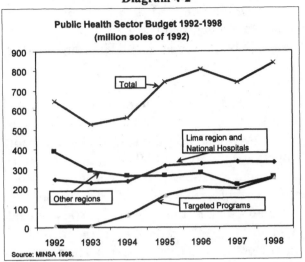

Diagram 4-2

While the institutional set-up remains unchanged, dissatisfaction with the role of the regions led the Government to seek to carry out new health activities through the development of targeted programs implemented by the regions, using funds transferred by MINSA and earmarked for specific activities. These programs (described below) have changed the balance of power in the sector. While the budget of the overall public health sector has grown considerably, the budget of the regions has fallen slightly in real terms (Diagram 4-2). As a proportion of the total budget, the weight of the regions has been halved from 60% in 1992 to 30% in 1998. On the other hand, the targeted programs have grown from 2% in 1992 to 30% in 1998.

NATIONAL HEALTH PROGRAMS OF MINSA

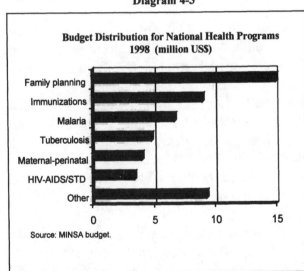

Diagram 4-3

The main unit of MINSA that deals with specific personal health services is the *Dirección General de Salud de las Personas* (DGSP). This unit is subdivided into 15 categorical programs (including four communicable disease, and eight demographic group programs). Some of these programs have a primarily normative and monitoring function while others are engaged in service provision. Some provide drugs and medical supplies. Some are directly in charge of the implementation of activities at a national level. Funding priority within DGSP is given to the National Family Planning Program, which has been assigned an independent budget since 1996 in an effort to boost its activities. Other major program priorities in descending order of budgetary allocation are immunizations, malaria, tuberculosis, maternal-perinatal health, and HIV-AIDS/STD (Diagram 4-3). *The Dirección General de Salud Ambiental* (DIGESA) also has national programs of relevance to the poor in the areas of Environmental Management (including water, food and animal management).

In addition to the <u>categorical</u> programs mentioned above, there exist a number of targeted programs that are specially financed and administered, with the objective of better targeting the poor. In some cases, the targeted programs finance activities of the categorical programs. The main such programs are listed below. The first two are the largest and are almost entirely funded by the public treasury. The three largest externally-funded programs are also described.

i. *Salud Básica,* with around US$100 million budgeted for 1998, was the first, and remains the largest, targeted support program.[23] It was started in 1994 with the objective of making the many health centers and health posts that were being rehabilitated by other projects operational. Its tightly-managed vertical administration was set up to by-pass the cumbersome public sector system and ensure swift disbursements and expense reporting. While it included some funds for infrastructure and equipment, these were never more than 10% of the investment. The largest expenditure is for the payment of health staff who are hired under a unique regimen of short-term contracts to work in underserved areas. Higher wages attract teams of physicians, nurses, professional midwives, dentists, and others to staff even isolated peripheral health facilities that never before had professional providers. Second in importance, one-third of the *Salud Básica* budget goes to drugs, supplies, training, supervision, and other operating expenses of the national health programs. *Salud Básica* also assigns 13% of its budget to finance the CLAS (described below). While *Salud Básica* emphasizes the 7 poorest departments (33% of its funds go to those departments which hold 22% of the population), all departments benefit from this program.

ii. PACFO (*Programa de Complementación Alimentaria para Grupos en Mayor Riesgo*) is managed by the *Instituto Nacional de Salud* (a decentralized agency of MINSA that functions autonomously) and channeled around US$24 million in 1998 for food supplements to five of the seven poorest departments, which were historically isolated from the main-stream economy of Peru and later suffered most under the struggle with the Shining Path terrorists. PACFO benefits are available to all children ages 6-36 months in these departments. Communities assign representatives to oversee distribution of the PACFO multi-grain fortified pre-cooked weaning food, which is done from health centers. These transfers account for a fourth of the total public health budget in those departments.[24]

iii. The large externally financed projects (which include the *Proyecto de Salud y Nutrición Básica* (PSNB), financed by World Bank; *Proyecto 2000*, financed by USAID; and the *Proyecto de Fortalecimiento de los Servicios de Salud* (PFSS

---

[23] It began life as part of a multiple-sector program to target public expenditures (*Programa de Focalización del Gasto Público*). This program later changed its name, reflecting a new focus that moved away from targeting the poor to making basic services available to all (*Programa de Salud Básica para Todos,* hereafter *Salud Básica*). This change in name seems to reflect both a change in the political mood and the technical realization, based on the early implementation of the program, that inclusion of the poor, while difficult to achieve, is an easier task than exclusion of the non-poor.

[24] PACFO is controversial. Critics argue that if the objective is preventing malnutrition, some resources should be applied to reaching pregnant women and that many non-poor children are receiving food unnecessarily. The INS claims that malnutrition among children in the PACFO departments has been falling at a rate 50% faster than the average decline in malnutrition among children in rural areas.

financed by IDB) are expected to make disbursements that add up to around $20 million to $25 million in 1999. The first two concentrate their investments in departments and provinces classified as poor, and are focused on strengthening intramural and extramural maternal and child health services. *Proyecto 2000* places more emphasis on maternal-reproductive health services than on child health services while PSNB focuses on both. Each of the two projects is developing its own health care delivery model through clinical and community volunteer training, IEC activities, and health service management improvement. PFSS, on the other hand, is not a service delivery project and is not targeted to poverty areas. Rather, it supports system-wide improvements in management training, health system support services (supervision and monitoring, information system, logistics, maintenance, and communication), equipment, and health sector reform studies.

TARGETING IN THE MINISTRY OF HEALTH

There has been much debate concerning the accuracy of the targeting by the targeted programs. Are they effectively directed to the poor? This section analyzes the regional distribution of the main MINSA-based programs according to departmental levels of poverty.[25] Departments were classified by MINSA following the poverty map used by the public sector in Peru into four groups: "very poor, poor, medium and acceptable". More sophisticated poverty maps have recently been developed by MINPRE and other public and private institutions, including measurement of intra-departmental poverty levels, but are still not widely used. The Department-based map continues in use by most public institutions and retains an intuitive appeal for public opinion that more sophisticated maps continue to lack.

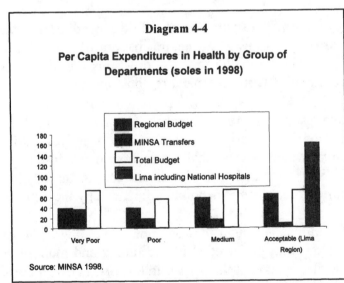

Diagram 4-4

Per Capita Expenditures in Health by Group of Departments (soles in 1998)

Source: MINSA 1998.

The degree to which expenditures are directed to the poor or rich Departments varies according to the channel of expenditures. Diagram 4-4 shows the per capita distribution of expenditures across the four groups of departments separating the "core" regional budget expenditures from the targeted program expenditures. Three clear patterns emerge. First, the regional budget is regressive. Per capita allocations assigned through regional budgets are higher in the richer departments. Per capita allocations in Lima (before including the budget of the National Hospitals which are mostly in Lima) are 66% higher than in the poorest departments.

---

[25] The data base was prepared by OGP (*Oficina General de Planificación*) for this study. It does not include health investments managed by other ministries.

By contrast, the targeted programs are fairly well targeted geographically. Per capita transfers to the poorest group of departments are 5 times larger than they are for Lima. The targeted programs account for almost half the public health spending in the poorest departments and for smaller proportions in the rest of the country. Although there are some transfers for Lima, these represent only a small fraction of the total. In per capita terms, transfers to the poorer departments double the national average and transfers to Lima are less than half the national average.

The targeted programs have different degrees of progressivity. Much of the regional progressivity is due to the presence of PACFO, which is entirely dedicated to the poorest departments and provides almost 40% of the transfers to those departments. Taken independently, *Salud Básica* is less progressive. *Salud Básica* contends that large numbers of the poor live in the richer regions and that the funds transferred to the richer regions are directed to the poorer districts within those regions. Data is not presently available to establish if that is being achieved.[26] Also, PACFO is only one of many food and nutrition programs by the Peruvian government. The overall distribution of food and nutrition programs is hard to establish but is believed to be regressive.

In the aggregate, in 1998 the pro-poor bias of the targeted programs could only compensate partially for the pro-rich bias of the core budget. Leaving aside the budget of the National Hospitals, per capita expenditures budgeted for 1998 were similar for the "very poor", "medium" and Lima Departments. A more detailed analysis shows that six of the poorer departments have total per capita spending higher than the national average. The only departments with even higher total spending per capita are those on the southern and eastern borders, usually considered to be of military interest.

Given the highly regressive starting point in the distribution of public expenditures, it has been difficult for the government to progress towards a neutral pattern of expenditure. While the amount of targeting incorporated into the targeted programs constitutes an important achievement, there remain significant problems and regional inequities:

- First and foremost, the targeted programs are *vulnerable to fiscal and political changes*. The "neutrality" achieved in the original 1998 budget was lost during execution of the budget. At mid-year there was a fiscal contraction in response to the effects of the Asian crisis. MINSA responded with significant cuts to the targeted programs which proved to be easier to cut than expenditures financed by the regional budget;
- The department-based poverty map is not enough for geographic targeting of health interventions. A more precise methodology is needed for designing and monitoring program targeting. In addition to the general poverty map indicators, MINSA needs indicators of burden of disease to guide its investments;

---

[26] *Salud Básica* originated as part of a "program for the targeting of public expenditures" that covered several ministries. Eventually become independent of that program and changed its name to "Basic Health for all." The new name may reflect a lesser emphasis on targeting.

- The achievement of equalizing expenditures across regions is dwarfed by a remaining inequity favoring Lima. The National Hospitals, most of which are in Lima, account for 24% of the total public health budget. This budget is in addition to th t of the Lima region. While the last few decades have seen an improved access to the specialized hospitals in Lima by non-Lima residents made possible by cheaper and faster transportation, and communications, these facilities continue to benefit the population of Lima to a greater extent than the population of the rest of the country;
- Finally, MINSA equalizes per capita spending for the population as a whole, but 26% of the population are affiliated to IPSS and should be excluded from MINSA's calculations. If the above calculation is done estimating MINSA per capita expenditures for the <u>uninsured</u> population (i.e., excluding the population affiliated to IPSS), a strong bias reappears in favor of the two richer groups of departments which contain only 44% of the uninsured population, but receive two thirds of MINSA's budget).

While the main form of targeting is geographic, the targeted programs are also benefiting the poor by focussing expenditures on communicable diseases. *Salud Básica* provides financing for the categoric disease-based programs. Funding for tuberculosis and malaria programs has grown by a multiple of 10 from 1992-3 to 1998. International studies show that this type of investment tends to be very pro-poor. As explained in chapter 2, communicable diseases are the cause of 45% of deaths among the poorest 20% and 22% among the richest 20%. Mortality rates are almost three times higher among the former compared with the latter. Hence, an accelerated decline in mortality from communicable disease distributed evenly across all social classes would benefit the poorest 20% almost 10 times as much as it would the richest 20%.

The targeted programs have clearly succeeded in expanding the geographical coverage of health services by making services available and improving their quality in remote locations. Chapter 1 shows that this has been beneficial to many of the poor. But it also shows how access by many of the poor remains limited. Chapter 4 analyzes the cost barrier.

PRODUCTIVITY IN PRIMARY HEALTH CLINICS

The efforts to increase the number of primary facilities have been successful, but they now create new challenges. Productivity in primary health clinics remains at very low levels and unit costs are very high. On average, health workers in MINSA (including clinical technicians) produce in the range of 288 to 738 consultations in a year, or roughly between 1 and 2 per day. The 1,020 health centers, usually employing 3-5 health professionals produce on average around 16 consultations per day. The 4,700 health posts on average produce around 3 consultations per day. These low averages disguise a high degree of dispersion. The majority of facilities are concentrated at extremely low productivity levels. 73% of MINSA health centers have 7 or less daily consultations per health professional. 70% of health posts have less than 3 consultations per health professional. As a point of comparison, a primary care physician in private practice in Lima or in a busy hospital can see around 40 patients in an afternoon. Low productivity translates into high unit costs: ambulatory consultations in primary clinics (56 soles) are more costly than ambulatory consultations in public hospitals (31 soles).[27] Productivity is slightly higher in urban areas, but even there the average is only 6 consultations/day per professional. When comparing groups of departments, productivity is slightly higher in Metropolitan Lima (7/day).

While there is no dispute about the existence of low levels of productivity in most health clinics, the figures quoted above exaggerate the problem because of three weaknesses in the data available: the 1996 Infrastructure Census (CISRESA 1996). First, this data base combines data on human resources for 1996 with production data for 1995 from the health information system. Using 1996 production data for *Salud Básica* facilities (which constituted a subset of the total) productivity increases by about 50% —higher, but still extremely low. Second, many of these facilities were recently rehabilitated and may have been in the process of initiating activities in 1995-96. Third, these productivity measures include only the production of clinical intramural contacts. Many facilities also produce preventive activities and extramural activities. *Salud Básica* has tried to measure these activities and estimates that *Salud Básica* staff produce almost 2 preventive activities per day and an average of almost one extramural consultation per day. While the definitions for non clinical activities are vague and the data are likely to underestimate the effort assigned to these activities, their inclusion does not change the basic picture of low levels of productivity.

A visit to most facilities confirms this picture. From health posts to hospitals, the entire sector seems caught in a marketing effort to attract a wider clientele. Early in the decade, the lack of demand was mainly blamed on key supply bottlenecks –shortages of inputs, frequent closings, short hours. Today these bottlenecks have largely been solved. While many local administrators think that their problem can be solved by further upgrading their facility, MINSA administrators are concerned about evidence of underutilized modern equipment.[28] The Government is planning to increase utilization by introducing *Seguros Públicos* (public insurance schemes described below) to increase demand by overcoming the economic barriers to access. It also plans to improve the quality of the service by improving incentives and management using a combination of new payment systems designed to finance outputs, rather than inputs, new management tools, greater autonomy, and greater participation of civil society in public service management. These reforms were pioneered by the creation of community-managed publicly financed health committees (CLAS). The government is considering an expansion of this experience. It is also considering the creation of autonomous networks of providers (*Redes*). The CLAS and the *Redes* are discussed below.

NEW INITIATIVES TO IMPROVE MANAGEMENT AND COMMUNITY PARTICIPATION

The CLAS (*Comités Locales de Administración de Salud*) are private, non-profit, community-administered institutions created by community members around a health

---

[27] This comparison excludes asset depreciation, which is substantially higher in hospitals.
[28] There is much anecdotal evidence of this. A study financed by the IDB will measure the utilization of the US$50 million worth of equipment purchased for first and second level facilities under the *Proyecto de Fortalecimiento de los Servicios de Salud*.

center or post. Their functions are to work with health providers to develop a local health plan, define the budget to implement the plan, and monitor expenditures and the provision of health services to the community. The objective of CLAS is to improve the quality and coverage of ambulatory services at the primary health level through greater participation by the community in planning, administration, management, and supervision of public resources. In December 1997, three years after the program's initiation, there were 548 CLAS formed in 26 of the 32 health regions or subregions.[29] These CLAS administered 611 health establishments, about 10 percent of those in the country, attending about 75% of the 2.65 million inhabitants in their area of jurisdiction, according to 1997 service data. A recent study comparing CLAS and non-CLAS establishments found that the CLAS have higher rates of community participation and have been quicker at introducing improvements to the service (Table 4-1).

Table 4-1

Improvements in Service Delivery in Community-Managed Publicly Financed Health Committee and Non-Community-Managed Publicly Financed Health Committee facilities

INDICATORS OF COMMUNITY PARTICIPATION IN CLAS AND NON-CLAS HEALTH SERVICES %	HEALTH CENTERS		HEALTH POSTS	
	CLAS	Non-CLAS	CLAS	Non-CLAS
	(n=5)	(n=15)	(n=14)	(n=32)
The community organization meets regularly	100	67	86	72
Meetings are led by a community member	100	60	93	88
Women participate in the community organization	100	80	93	88
Women participate in training and decision-making	100	67	86	72
Disadvantaged groups are adequately represented	60	33	29	41
Needs of socially and economically disadvantaged groups are addressed in the local health plan	100	87	86	66
The community approves paid health personnel	60	7	43	22
The community evaluates personnel or the local health Program	40	13	57	28
Indicators of Improvements in Services %:				
Needed services are newly available	80	47	86	53
Clinic hours, waiting time is improved	100	73	86	75
A health promoter program was implemented	80	60	71	50
More extramural activities and home visits	100	80	86	91
Community projects have been successful	80	33	57	50

Note: Proportion of health facilities that satisfy selected indicators of community participation, based on subjective rating by health personnel in each facility, by type of health facility.
Source: Data collected by J. Salcedo from 66 low-income urban health facilities, Region of Arequipa – Peru for the Programa de Fortalecimiento de Servicios de Salud; data analysis by L. Altobelli (1998).

The CLAS is constituted by six members of the community plus the director of the health facility who serves as manager of the CLAS. Under Peruvian law, these entities are allowed to receive public funds to produce services specified by a three year contract. Under the contract, management of the facilities is officially transferred by MINSA to the CLAS. MINSA finances the CLAS through transfers and through direct payment of some of the staff.[30] This arrangement has a number of important advantages:

---

[29] No permits for the formation of new CLAS were issued in 1998, at the time of writing this report government officials informed the Bank that new permits would be issued shortly.
[30] Two groups of staff exist; those who already had a civil service contract when the CLAS was formed are paid directly by MINSA; the majority are hired and paid by the CLAS.

- *Improved planning of health activities*. All CLAS prepare annual Local Health Plans (LHP), which are based on a diagnosis of the actual population size, socio-demographic characteristics, health status, and major causes of morbidity and mortality. The LHP sets targets, activities and the required budgets to implement those activities. It is approved by the Board of the CLAS and is the basis of the performance contract signed with regional health authorities. CLAS undertake an annual local census as part of the community diagnosis to prepare the LHP;
- *Improved incentives to raise productivity and improved accountability*. The contract between CLAS and MINSA is designed to finance outputs rather than inputs. The CLAS is held accountable for reaching the targets agreed on in the LHP and presenting audited financial and technical reports related to the management of funds;
- *Flexibility in the management of budgets*. CLAS are not subject to the slow procedures of public sector budget management and procurement regulations. Most health centers cannot manage public funds (these are managed by the health regions), CLAS by contrast can do so with great agility;
- *Flexibility in the hiring of staff*. CLAS hire staff under private sector legislation. The use of short-term contracts and bonuses provide them with a strong incentive framework;
- *Improved quality of care*. The CLAS members are empowered to demand better treatment of clients and oversee the purchase of necessary equipment and supplies to improve health care provision.

The CLAS system has been received with great sympathy by communities, but has encountered significant resistance within the public sector since 1997. MINSA has refused to issue any new permits for the creation of new CLAS, despite the existence of numerous requests. This resistance is mainly based on concern by Regional health officials with the loss of direct control over health facilities and staff. Health professionals who work for the CLAS are often supportive, but would like to enjoy greater stability and higher benefits. Public sector unions which represent the shrinking fraction of staff with civil service contracts, view the system as a threat.

The initial years of experience with CLAS revealed a number of weaknesses, many of which are now being addressed.

- CLAS worked better in the less-poor urban communities, where users can afford higher co-payments and require less exceptions from payment and where a higher formal education facilitates the development of management skills in the community. Co-payments supplementing government transfers are utilized to contract more health personnel, update physical facilities, and purchase equipment and supplies. The presence of community members with skills in management and accounting is another factor that contributes to the success of CLAS. These factors, which are generally not present in rural and very low-income areas, should now be taken into consideration when planning support for CLAS. Plans to provide higher transfers and management training to CLAS members in poor undeveloped areas should also be developed;

- There had been no systematic evaluations of the CLAS program to investigate its impact on coverage, quality and opportunity of services, and community satisfaction. Several small studies have now been carried out and a new major study on CLAS is in the final stages of completion, with preliminary results showing improved client satisfaction and increased utilization of CLAS facilities as compared to non-CLAS facilities;
- There was no mechanism established to monitor progress on the health targets of the management contracts. Supervision was mainly focused on financial and legal procedures. Now, a more streamlined method for estimating budgets on the basis of the LHP has been issued and could also facilitate evaluation of results, potentially strengthening the LHP as a management instrument. Health regions have mainly focused on controlling the CLAS. There are now plans to develop capacity in the regions to provide technical support for the implementation of the LHP. This will be done sometimes directly by the regions, and at others by recruiting specialized services of NGOs;
- While there are no known instances of open corruption, there have been cases where audits have identified the use of incorrect financial procedures. More training and orientation of CLAS members is expected to correct those problems.

Parallel to expanding the CLAS, MINSA is considering the creation of *Redes* – autonomous networks of health providers for the first and second level of health care. The *Redes* would build on the experience of autonomy of the CLAS. Their larger size would allow them to benefit from economies of scale and from more sophisticated management. Also, greater efficiency could be obtained from referral and counter-referral of patients. The proposal includes the development of new payment mechanisms. Some key questions are still under consideration:

- What is the future role of the regional health authorities? Will they retain administrative functions (such as the management of human resources), or will they be limited to a normative role? If the regions do not disappear and new layers are created to manage the networks and to 'purchase services', there is a risk of creating new layers of bureaucracy;
- How will the vitality achieved by the CLAS be preserved? Their virtue to date has been the great independence they enjoy for the programming of activities, budgetary management and local level participation. If the CLAS become a part of the *Redes* and are operated under external authority (in the same way as any other health center), there is a risk that their vitality could become stifled by bureaucracy. An alternative for consideration would be to retain the autonomy of the CLAS and to establish voluntary forms of association that would force the *Redes* to demonstrate that they can provide advantages such as improved management, technical assistance, and lower prices for the purchase of inputs.

CLAS is a unique experience for the health sector in Peru, but is not the only program of its type to incorporate community control of public services management. The concept of civil participation in efforts to eradicate poverty has been empirically tested with sufficient frequency to confirm its validity as a critical element for the sustainability of social development programs. The internationally-acclaimed experience of *Villa El Salvador* in self-management (*auto-gestión*) is a prime example close to home. Other examples in urban development, the education sector, and micro-enterprise development show further proof of the improved efficiency obtained from public investment within the framework of public sector-community collaboration. Three country experiences in the region, aside from Peru, with participation of civil society in health service delivery are discussed in Box 4-2.

Box 4-2

Participation by Civil Society in Health Services: Experience of Three Other Latin American Countries

Lessons learned from civil society participation in the health sector center around how social control leads to improvements in quality of services and quality of expenditures, which in turn promotes increased utilization of services with results of lowering of unit costs. Each of the following country experiences has a distinct organizational and financial framework, but with the common element of social control over public services:

Venezuela*- Under decentralized health sector reform in 1990, the State of Lara created a public institution, Fundasalud, to channel Ministry of Health funds to eligible NGOs (now over 600 total) under contract to manage public health services, including 60 ambulatory health centers, various hospitals, milk distribution programs, and others. Most participating NGOs are health committees legally constituted as "civil associations", or "neighbors associations" (operating mostly in rural areas since the 1970s). The NGOs administer public funds and serve as watch dogs to ensure quality of care and efficiency. An evaluation comparing Fundasalud ambulatory health centers with traditionally state-managed ones showed significantly better client perceptions of quality of medical, nursing, dental, laboratory, and emergency services; significantly higher rating of the operation of the centers; and significantly greater demand for services resulting in lower costs per client, as shown.

VENEZUELA	6 health facilities with civil participation	6 health facilities without civil participation
Average total cost per month	2,928,832 Bs.	2,336,833 Bs.
Average number of patients per month	1,730	423
Average cost per patient	1,693 Bs.	5,524 Bs.

Source: Data adapted from C. Mascareño (1997).

Colombia+- Under the 1993 health reform, all Colombians are required to select an "*entidad promotora de salud*" (EPS) that administers the pre-paid insurance policies of its affiliates. For 12 million persons unable to buy insurance, qualified beneficiaries select an "*administrador del régimen subsidiado*" (ARS) which function as state-reimbursed EPS. The very poorest segment of the population participates in an extended version of ARS called "*empresas solidarias de salud*" (ESS) that have two peculiarities: (1) they are *owned* by the subsidized beneficiaries, and (2) they function in areas where other ARS have no interest in entering. ESS are initiated through a multi-stage process of community orientation, health and business management training; self-elected community groups become private health cooperatives which contract with the government and sub-contract to private or public providers.

COLOMBIA - Rural Access	*Empresas Solidarias de Salud* (ESS)	Other ARS
Have own network of primary care	95.0%	63.5%
Contract with public hospitals	95.0%	87.3%
Contract with private clinics	51.6%	46.8%
Rural coverage with own teams	60.0%	9.5%

Source: Reunirse, Cider, Universidad de Los Andes. In: F. Perez Calle (1998).

> **Brazil++** - The small fishing and agricultural municipality of Icapuí in northeast Brazil has implemented an experience in community participation whereby the municipality manages health facilities, health providers are contracted by the government, and the population pays no fees for health care. The community contributes to health services planning and evaluation through open-air meetings and other community assemblies. Recently, some Brazilian states are transferring administration of large hospitals to "*Organizaciones Sociales*", comprised of civil servants, justice system representatives, NGOs, and public administration directors. The hope is that co-management of the more expensive and complex services will increase production, reduce costs, and improve the relationship between health workers and their clients.

Sources: *Carlos Mascareño, "Ambulatory health centers with citizen participation, promoted by FUNDASALUD in the State of Lara – Venezuela", Prepared for IDB seminar on *Social Programs, Poverty and Citizen Participation*, Cartagena. Colombia, March 12-13, 1998.

+Francisco Pérez, "*Participación comunitaria en la producción y provisión de bienes públicos: Análisis comparativo de las Empresas Solidarias de Salud de Colombia y los centros ambulatorios de Fundasalud en Venezuela*", Prepared for the IDB seminar on *Social Programs, Poverty and Citizen Participation*, Cartagena. Colombia, March 12-13, 1998.

++ Carlos Komora, "El control social como factor de mejora de la gestión de los sistemas locales de salud; el Sistema Local de Salud de Icapuí, Ceará, Brasil", Prepared for IDB seminar on *Social Programs, Poverty and Citizen Participation*, Cartagena. Colombia, March 12-13, 1998.

EQUITY AND EFFICIENCY IN PUBLIC HOSPITALS

Public hospitals are an important part of the public health sector in terms of resources consumed and of services produced. They absorb about 55% of the public health budget, and produce about half of ambulatory consultations, most high-cost interventions and practically all inpatient services.[31] In recent years, hospitals have received a small fraction of public investment as MINSA and external financiers have emphasized investments in ambulatory clinics.[32] Hospitals can play an important role in providing the population, and especially the poor, with an implicit form of insurance against catastrophic events in countries with underdeveloped insurance systems. The uninsured must often meet the financial burden of medical emergencies through debt, distress sales of real assets, or reductions in food or other important consumption items. A growing number of studies suggest that worsened health, because of the high cost of medical care and lost income, often forces people into poverty.[33] Others suggest the poor may suffer most from these events.[34]

While benefits channeled by public hospitals are greater for the rich than they are for the poor, it would be wrong to conclude that hospitals play no role for the poor. MINSA hospital services are crucial for the poor who have few alternative options for secondary-level services. For the whole of the population, MINSA provides 65% of inpatient services. For the poorest 20% MINSA provides 85% of these services –three quarters of that through hospitals and the rest through health clinics. While in recent years it may have been valid for policy-makers to emphasize the development of preventive and ambulatory services based on primary care clinics, in future the key distinction that needs to be made is not between primary health clinics and hospitals. It is between basic

---

[31] The relative cost of hospitals is an update of estimates from Francke 1997; p. 34.

[32] There have been a few large investments in Specialized Institutes. The IDB-financed "Fortalecimiento de losservicios de salud" project may also have allocated a third of the $45 million of medical equipment purchased to secondary hospitals.

[33] Gwatkin (forthcoming).

[34] Hammer (1999).

services –some of which need to be provided by hospitals—and high-tech services. Emphasis should also be directed to increasing the access of the poor to hospital services.

There are two significant problems with public hospitals. First, while they are practically the only source of secondary and tertiary services for the poor, they assign only a small fraction of their resources to serve the poor. This is mainly due to a high degree of commercialization, and lack of regulation. Second, there are problems of internal efficiency, as most hospitals are hugely underutilized. This section discusses these features. Recommendations for further reforms are to be found in Chapter 8.

Autonomy, Distorted Subsidies and Inefficiency in Allocation

Several countries attempting to modernize their public sectors through market-oriented reforms strive to give greater autonomy to their public hospitals. Peruvian hospitals, by contrast, already enjoy a large amount of autonomy (see Box 4-3). This autonomy is underpinned by a rare privilege in the public administration, and one forbidden to most ambulatory care clinics: hospitals have independent budgets and the authority to spend them.[35] What makes the independent budgets relevant is the existence of large revenues from co-payments by users ("own resources"). Revenues from tariffs have become a growing fraction of the budget of most hospitals. For the National Hospitals in Lima, these revenues constituted 6%-7% of the total in the early 1980s, grew to almost 10% in 1992, and constitute at least 25% of the total today (Table 4-2).[36] The budget paid by the treasury pays for the payroll and some of the fixed costs of running the hospital. "Own resources" pay for all discretional spending. Through the use of these funds, the hospital gets to decide what to produce, who to produce it for, and how to spend its revenues. In Lima, own revenues pay for over half of goods and services and for almost all the investment, giving the hospital enormous leverage to decide what to produce.[37] MINSA plays no role in approving these investments, so hospitals decide what niche to enter with great autonomy. Some of the hospital revenues are paid to the hospital staff, circumventing the prohibition to top up salaries of public employees, through the use of a wide variety of benefits. These include study grants for hospital administrators (a significant number of administrators of national hospitals have gained access to ESAN's reputable Master in Hospital Administration

Table 4-2

Revenues from Tariffs in Lima Hospitals

Type of Hospital	Revenues from tariffs as percentage of total budget	Revenues from tariffs as percentage of expenditures on	
		Goods and services	Capital Investment
National Hospitals	23%	53%	99%
Specialized Institutes	26%	50%	71%
Other Lima Hospitals	18%	61%	100%

Source: OGP.

---

[35] Health Centers, many of which today may be more complex than some hospitals, do not have spending authority. The CLAS receive spending authority. For the Clinics, this is an important motivation to change their status into CLAS. For the local health authorities, this is a reason to oppose their conversion.

[36] Estimates from ANSSA for the early 1980s (quoted by Iglesias (1993)); Iglesias (1993) for 1992 and OGP for 1997.

[37] With the exception of one large investment financed by the Government for Lima's Cancer hospital.

course) or productivity bonuses, or food baskets for workers. These revenues are also important to undertake investments in high-tech equipment that provides a gratification to the hospital staff in the form of more rewarding professional work.

Box 4-3

The Origins of Autonomy for Hospital Managers

Until the 1960s, the most important hospitals in Peru were run by local charities, often with support from other local institutions such as religious congregations, local authorities and universities. These hospitals were nationalized by General Velazco's administration in the early 1970s and turned into "National Hospitals." Their staff became public employees and the role of all other institutions in the governance of the hospitals was eliminated.[38] MINSA had never managed to set policies, plan or regulate the simpler hospitals built during the 1960s and it never developed the tools for the more complex role of regulating a hugely enlarged hospital sector. As a result, hospital directors (usually a physician operating with the advice of the other senior physicians in the hospital) made decisions with little guidance from MINSA or from local authorities. This established a tradition of great autonomy for hospital managers. As the National Hospitals include most teaching hospitals, this tradition has now been extended to all public hospitals. Autonomy was enhanced by the steep increase in user fees that accompanied the fiscal crisis of the late 1980s.

Under-utilization of Hospitals

There is a problem of misalignment between the capital structure (physical plant and technology) and the actual services provided by hospitals, as unmet needs and congestion of some services in some hospitals coexist with a surprisingly low level of hospital bed utilization. Nationally, only 52% of bed-days are utilized. For comparison purposes, an 80% occupancy rate is often perceived as a threshold of concern in the USA; the rate of occupancy of all public hospitals in Honduras is 70%. The degree of under-utilization varies by category of hospital and by location and is highest outside the three main cities (Table 4-3). Much of the under-utilization arises from duplication: MINSA's underutilized hospitals stand side-by-side with IPSS underutilized hospitals in 20 departmental capitals; 11 of these also have a military or police hospital. An experiment to reduce duplication by the joint utilization of facilities by MINSA and IPSS beneficiaries was conducted in a dozen hospitals starting in the mid-1980s, and is in the process of being dismantled today. The experiment was poorly designed and received no technical assistance. No system was ever designed for the joint utilization of facilities. Instead ad-hoc arrangements were established in each hospital, unaccompanied by any attempt to cost and price services, or to monitor the stream of benefits for users of each sub-sector.

Table 4-3

Bed Occupancy Rate (% of available bed-days utilized in 1995)

	MINSA	IPSS	Military/ Police	Private
National Hospitals	60	78	69	21
Other Hospitals	31	45	25	21
Health Centers	9	11	15	7

Source: CISRESA 1996 (Internet version); utilization data for 1995.

---

[38] These nationalized hospitals were added to the fairly large number of new hospitals built during the 1960s.

This independence in decision making has created a situation of "micro-economic efficiency", where hospital administrators respond to market signals, but some of these signals are distorted and create problems of overall allocative efficiency (Box 4-4). The management objective is to find ways to transform the subsidies received from the state —in the form of assets and the fixed payroll— into cash. This often provides incentives for activities that are not central to and may even distract resources from the "mission" of the hospitals. Outpatient primary services are profitable in the sense of providing net cash income to the hospital and hospitals make evident efforts to increase their production of these services, even if the overall cost of producing the services at the hospital level is higher than the cost of the same service in a clinic. Despite the large investments in MINSA ambulatory clinics, MINSA hospitals defended "their market share" and increased their production of ambulatory consultations by 55% between 1994 and 1997. Signs of entrepreneurship abound in the best-managed hospitals. Many hospitals have opened outpatient services, in the afternoon and the evening, hiring young private doctors who are paid an agreed fraction of the revenue they generate for the hospital. Some hospitals have made significant investments in improving outpatient facilities in an effort to attract patients from the competition (often private clinics from across the street). Some, such as Arzobispo Loayza, have built private wings within the hospital's premises where patients pay higher tariffs in exchange for better accommodation, easier access to senior physicians, and shorter waiting periods for busy high-end technology. Outside Lima, some hospitals allow the use of some of their facilities for the treatment of private patients ("out of hours", sometimes in exchange for a symbolic payment to the hospital). In some cases, the kitchen or the laundry staff are allowed to use the facilities for outside business.

Box 4-4

Allocative Costs of Unregulated Hospital Autonomy

- Hospital administrators take only cash flows into account. Costs, such as salaries paid directly by the treasury, are not included in these calculations;
- Partly as a result of the above, maintenance is neglected. The administrators impute no value to the use of the asset stock they manage and this constitutes a giant subsidy to the hospitals (many of the older hospitals occupy huge tracts of prime real estate). The autonomization of hospitals in the UK set a large minimum return to assets standard—profits could only be declared after that level of revenues was achieved;
- Private clinics complain that hospitals compete under unfair conditions: in addition to receiving subsidies, hospitals often pay no taxes for their privatized services;
- Hospitals are geared to compete with, rather than to complement, the rest of the health care network. Ambulatory primary care is often more profitable than first and second level inpatient services; hence hospitals compete for patients for the former, but make no efforts to attract mothers for birth deliveries or to reduce congestion and increase user satisfaction with emergency services. High complexity facilities accept and encourage profitable, low-complexity patients, even if by doing this they create congestion that limits access to more costly patients. This system provides no incentive for the development of "gatekeepers" or for the establishment of systems of referral or counter-referral;
- Medium-cost investments are based on the willingness to pay of the wealthier users. High cost investments in complex technology depend on the availability of grants (e.g. by Rotaries, bilateral donors or Regional Governments) or on provider loans. The poor get no vote and national criteria of

need or burden of disease have no way to influence investments in hospitals;

- Lack of regulation by Ministry programs. The Ministry has no instrument to enforce regulations. Hospitals do not use official MINSA care protocols, do not participate in training programs, are not subject to supervision visits from MINSA program officials, and often do not provide required statistics;
- Hospitals have no incentive to do prevention work. MINSA has no prevention program for chronic disease.

Most important of all, the existing system of unregulated autonomy provides no incentives for the hospital to serve the poor.

5. REFORMS IN FINANCING OF SERVICES

THE ECONOMIC BARRIER

The cost of medical attention is a deterrent for the poor. Labor costs, which are paid by the Treasury, tend to be moderately to strongly subsidized by MINSA establishments. By contrast, most drugs and medical inputs, which are financed by the establishment out of revenues from user charges, are charged to the user at full cost plus a mark-up. Consequently, tariffs for services in public establishments are generally affordable. Drugs and medical inputs on the other hand constitute 71% of direct health expenditures. Among the poorest 20%, these items represent 81% of direct expenditures (Table 5-1). The poor make proportionately less use of inpatient services than they do for outpatient services. This again is likely to be partly an effect of the cost of inputs and transport. When all costs are included, the full cost of a normal birth delivery at a public hospital can reach $100, the full cost of a cesarean or a hernia operation can reach $400, whereby the cost of the tariff for the service may be no more than 10% of these totals.

Table 5-1

Out-of-pocket Health Expenditures by Quintile

	Total	Q1	Q2	Q3	Q4	Q5
Health Expenditures (soles per capita)	90	21	45	74	93	216
Of which (% distribution):	100	100	100	100	100	100
Outpatient Services	16	16	14	15	15	18
Inpatient Services	3	1	2	4	3	3
Diagnostic Analysis	10	3	7	10	8	12
Drugs and Inputs	71	80	77	71	74	67

Source: ENNIV 1997-Cuánto S.A.

Most MINSA facilities make an attempt to address the economic barriers to health care for the poor by reducing tariffs. Total exemptions from payment are rare —less than a fifth of the poor are exempt from payment for outpatient services and only a fourth of the poor are exempt from payment for inpatient services. However, many more among the poor (50%-66%) benefit from low or reduced payments in what is often regarded as a morally and financially more acceptable mechanism. Hospitals tend to be less generous than primary care clinics.[39]

The existing system of exceptions has several defects. First, there is no fund to subsidize drugs and inputs at the provider level. Most drugs dispensed are purchased by the provider and sold to the user at cost with a mark-up.[40] All revenues from the pharmacy are maintained in a separate account used only to restock inventories. Years of scarcity and high inflation rates have led to the development of a culture that places great store by protecting the integrity of these "rotating funds". Hence all exceptions are discouraged. Exceptions are also discouraged to protect a simple rule that provides transparency and

---

[39] Hospitals keep their revenues, while primary clinics share them with the regional office –this may explain the greater generosity found in clinics.
[40] The National Categoric Programs (described in Chapter 3) finance a few drugs (e.g. for malaria and tuberculosis); these are purchased by each region and distributed free of charge to the provider, who passes them on at no charge to the user.

accountability: only one person has the key to the pharmacy and all drugs dispensed have a cash entry counterpart. Any loss to the rotating fund is the responsibility of the person in charge of the pharmacy.

Second, exceptions for the poor have to be financed by local generosity, as there is no instrument to have subsidies "follow the poor". There is no national or regional or even municipal pool to subsidize establishments that receive large proportions of the poor. Each establishment finances the lost revenues from its own resources, even if some establishments serve a very poor constituency while others serve a richer population.[41] Many providers seem to set aside 10-20% of their revenues from tariffs for the poor. In the establishments serving a large proportion of the poor, this is not enough to cover all those that would need the subsidy. While most establishments may assign a fraction of funds to reduce co-payments by the poor, this is a voluntary decision taken mainly by the management of the facility. There is no obligation to do this. There is a growing concern that some of the more entrepreneurial establishments discourage use by the poor and may assign much less from their revenues for this purpose. This is believed to include some of the best National Hospitals and Institutes, which are moving to serve more of the middle class.

Third, there are no standard criteria or methodology to identify the poor. Each establishment develops its own system and applies it erratically most of the time. This, compounded by the greater influence and contacts of the middle class, partly explains why much of this subsidy gets diverted to the non poor: around half of the exemptions and reduced rates are captured by the richer 60% of households (Francke 1994).

THE PUBLIC INSURANCE SCHEMES

The government is beginning to confront the economic barrier with the introduction of schemes designed to provide universal access by vulnerable demographic groups to key services. The *Seguro Escolar* (insurance for schoolchildren) was created in 1997. It is now considering the creation of a *Seguro Materno Infantil* following the new international evidence on the benefits of such schemes; for example the hugely successful Bolivian scheme increased institutional coverage of births by 32% in only 18 months (see Box 5-1). Both schemes eliminate co-payments by patients at the point of use of the service and cover prescription drugs. A predefined package of services is provided to any member of an easily identifiable demographic group, and the government reimburses providers for these services. The *Seguro Escolar* is free of charge to beneficiaries. The Government is considering a small subsidized insurance premium (possibly free of charge in the poorest regions) for the SMI. The Government is also considering the creation of a scheme to target benefits to all individuals identified as poor.

---

[41] In theory, subregional offices pool all revenues from health centers and health posts and distribute them back according to need. In practice, this happens in few places, and even in those places, the funds pooled are redistributed mainly in proportion to revenue-collected and not to "need" (after taxing away a large slice for administrative expenses).

Box 5-1

Bolivia's Public Mother and Child Insurance

The Seguro Nacional de Maternidad y Niñez was created in 1996 as a complement to the decentralization of health services that had taken place a few months before. The decentralization transferred the responsibilities for all social services to regions and municipalities, and assigned them a global budget to cover these responsibilities. For health, the management of public clinics and hospitals was assigned to municipalities. Initially the health services were underfinanced, as municipalities assigned the budget to other more politically visible activities outside the health sector. The Seguro was created, after a process of consensus building and cajoling, to earmark part (3.2%) of the global budget targeted to municipalities to financing key services in health.

During its experience with hyperinflation in the 1980s, Bolivia allowed its public health providers to substantially increase tariffs from users of health services. The Seguro eliminated these tariffs and created a system of reimbursements for key services offered to mothers and children. Its principal objective was to increase coverage of services for mothers and children to reduce infant and maternal mortality. Funding for the Seguro is transferred by the treasury to municipal special accounts created especially for that purpose. Facilities present invoices for eligible services provided. These invoices are approved by a body that includes community representation. Once they are approved, the municipality makes a reimbursement from the special account. Important lessons emerge from the Bolivian experience:

- Comparing 1995 and 1997, a sample of public and private establishments showed an aggregate increase in coverage of 32% for institutional births, 45% for new ante-natal visits, and 70% for all antenatal visits.
- The package was provided free of cost at all levels of attention and at the establishments of the Ministry of Health and the Social Insurance (which are regarded as better quality). Services of the private sector were not reimbursed. This produced a number of significant shifts in demand: users switched from private to public producers (the increase in institutional births in public facilities was almost 50%, while births in private facilities fell by a third); from primary clinics to hospitals (two thirds of the increase was in third-level facilities); and initially from the Ministry to the social security facilities – until the latter began to refuse to provide services for the Seguro.
- Insurance covers only part of the inputs and provides no reimbursement for labor or other costs and payments are often made in kind, instead of cash. This has generated bottlenecks as providers find no incentive to meet the increase in demand, and the in-kind payments create rigidities and delays.

The government is preparing to launch a second generation of the Seguro (the Seguro Básico) aiming to confront the problems mentioned above and to increase coverage of key interventions. The new scheme would also attempt to create incentives for preventive and extramural activities.

The Seguro Escolar and the Seguro Materno Infantil. The *Seguro Escolar*, with a budget of about US$30 million for 1998 is designed to cover health services and drugs for all children aged 3-17 who attend public schools (around 6 million). During 1998, the scheme covered 4 million consultations. Although there is no systematic study to establish how much of this is a net increase in coverage, many hospitals are reporting higher attendance by children. Also, lower level facilities are reporting lower attendance as some users have switched into hospitals. The scheme suffers from logistic problems which need to be addressed to avoid the development of bottlenecks. Facilities complain that reimbursements are slow, and that they have been forced to cover many expenses from their own revenues. These problems arise from lack of clarity about what interventions are covered by the *Seguro Escolar,* and from the use of cumbersome and slow barter mechanisms for reimbursements —facilities are paid in inputs, instead of in cash. The main problem is that only the cost of inputs is reimbursed, whereas the revenues from tariffs, that existed before the *Seguro* was established, also covered other costs, including benefits for the staff (such as food baskets). This problem could become a true disincentive for the provision of services.

The proposed *Seguro Materno Infantil* (SMI) would cover a package of basic services for mothers and for children under 3 years of age (those between 3 and 17 are covered by the *Seguro Escolar*). The Seguro will cover outpatient consultations, inpatient stays, surgery, drugs and emergencies for a carefully chosen group of cost-effective interventions. The SMI would reimburse the facilities for services and inputs that would be provided without cost to the user. A pilot scheme is being implemented in two regions to test logistics and procedures, and to experiment with new payment mechanisms. The Government plans to introduce the SMI as a separate scheme. Once it has taken hold, it would establish a single public insurance consolidating it with the *Seguro Escolar* and possibly incorporating the option of using private providers.

A data base of poor households? While the *Seguros* would go a long way to surmount the economic barrier for mothers, infants and schoolchildren, it would not solve the problem of access to other hospital services by the poor. MINSA has been considering the creation of a system that would allow it to pay subsidies for catastrophic events only for the poor. A number of steps have already been taken to develop such a system, including the design and pilot testing of questionnaires and the statistical analysis of variables that could be used in an index to identify the poor. Two options under examination include an ambitious proposal to create a national or regional data base of the poor; and a modest proposal to use questionnaires, statistics and algorithms to improve and systematize the ways in which health facilities decide whom to exempt.

While the modest proposal is clearly workable, the Colombian experience (which inspired the ambitious proposal) suggests that the creation of a data base should not be undertaken in the short run: (i) To effectively reach the poor, the system needs to go beyond the facility and undertake a quasi-census approach —this would be costly and demanding; (ii) Several studies show that a large fraction of the poor in Peru move in and out of poverty every year; this implies that the data base would need to be updated periodically, adding substantially to the administrative costs; (iii) The experience of Colombia and other countries is that there is a great risk of political manipulation of the information. Once people understand how the classification is arrived at, many give false information to obtain the subsidy. Developing safeguards to limit this behavior adds to administrative costs; (iv) The population moves rapidly; in Colombia, after three years a third of the poor have moved; (v) Finally, qualified people are needed at the facility level to manage the data base; in Colombia it has been very hard to train and retain these people. Finally, despite the investment, there is no evidence to show that the system has substantially improved targeting in Colombia.

So far this report has focused on health service provision and financing. In the next two chapters, we look at the planning, management, and information systems needed to enhance the Ministry of Health's ability to orchestrate the reforms, and at the human resources required to implement them.

6. STRENGTHENING PLANNING, MANAGEMENT AND INFORMATION SYSTEMS IN THE MINISTRY OF HEALTH

MINSA'S ability to successfully prioritize and deliver health services to the poor is curtailed by inefficiencies in policy-setting and regulation. Fragmentation of its policy-setting function is one problem. It is compounded, however, by another: weak information systems. This section discusses these two deficiencies and describes the attempts underway to correct them.

FRAGMENTATION OF POLICYMAKING AND REGULATORY FUNCTIONS

Much fragmentation and duplication exist within MINSA. The problem is especially acute for interventions in maternal and child health (MCH), nutrition, and environmental health, none of which has a clear structure for policy or planning. In theory, MCH policy and planning is one of many responsibilities of the *Dirección General de Salud de las Personas (DGSP)*. Within DGSP, this responsibility is split into 8 national programs (for immunizations, child growth and development, diarrhea and cholera, acute respiratory infections, maternal-perinatal health, family planning, school-age/adolescent health, micronutrient deficiency prevention, and HIV-AID/STD), which are spread among various dependencies of DGSP. Two large and many small externally financed projects also finance MCH activities. Each of these projects are "vertically integrated": they have independent planning offices and each has components of institutional development (policy design, health sector financing, information systems), components to develop health care "software" (typically development of medical protocols and training, sometimes IEC) and components to invest in "hardware" for the public network (mostly equipment, in a few cases also construction). In environmental health, there are overlaps and often duplications in food quality control (DIGESA, INS and the municipalities duplicate actions in some areas and leave many areas uncovered) and vector control (DIGESA, INS, DGSP). In nutrition, overlap in functions occurs between DGSP, INS and many other public and private sector institutions outside MINSA (see Table 6-1).

Table 6-1

Fragmentation of Nutrition Programs

	Policy setting (P) Implementation [training, IEC, purchasing, etc.] (I) Monitoring & evaluation (ME)
Maternal-fetal nutrition	DGSP: Maternal-Perinatal (P, I, ME); Micronutrients (P, I, ME) INS/CENAN (P, I, ME)
Infant-child nutrition	DGSP: Micronutrients (P, I, ME); GM (P, I, ME); CDD (P, I); ARI (P, I) INS/CENAN (P, I, ME)
School-age/Adolescent nutrition	DGSP: School-age/Adolescent Health (P, I, ME) INS/CENAN (P, I, ME)
Micronutrients	DGSP: Micronutrients (P, I, ME); Maternal-Perinatal (P, I, ME) INS/CENAN (P, I, ME)
Food fortification	DGSP: Micronutrients (P, I, ME) INS/CENAN (P, I, ME)
Nutritional surveillance	INS/CENAN (P, I, ME)

Food programs	INS/CENAN (P, I, ME)
	Other sectors:
	   PROMUDEH-PRONAA (P, I, ME)
	   MINPRE-FONCODES (P, I, ME)
	   Municipalities (P, I, ME)
	   Private sector (P, I, ME)

Proper nutrition cannot be underestimated as the primary factor contributing to adequate growth and development of the individual as well as prevention or amelioration of infectious and chronic disease. As a component of maternal and child health, nutrition is primordial. Its poor status is also an accepted poverty indicator. These facts are recognized in the prevailing MINSA general policy document*, but are not translated into accommodation of the organizational framework to ensure that the appropriate actions are taken in extreme poverty populations at high nutritional risk. The table in this box makes it clear that nutrition is the domain of everyone, and of no one. The results are duplications and inconsistencies, and therefore inefficiencies, in both policy making and implementation. Nutrition is managed as an "add-on" to various health facility-based services, with no framework for integrated community prevention strategies. With no one concerned about the whole picture, many cracks are left and the poor fall between the cracks.

The nutrition scenario is complicated by food programs, which utilize the lion's share of nutrition resources and are dispersed among myriad public and private sector institutions. MINSA is responsible for 10-15% of the total country budget for food programs. Nearly all food programs outside the health sector are implemented without nutritional objectives (though school breakfast programs accounting for one quarter of all food programs are well justified because of their impact on educational objectives). Within MINSA, two food programs account for approximately 90% of the budget used for nutrition activities, but the larger of them is not focalized on segments of the population living in extreme poverty and both have weak community nutrition education components.

Source: *El Desafío del Cambio de Milenio: Un Sector Salud con Equidad, Eficiencia y Calidad – Lineamientos de Política de Salud 1995-2000*, Lima, Peru: *Ministerio de Salud*. 1995.

In MCH, there have been attempts to create "Coordination Committees" for specific topics, but, lacking a clear line of authority in charge of policy, these committees have become a meeting ground for project-financed consultants with no access to the political decision-makers. The only effective form of coordination has been the division of the country assigning regions to specific projects (there are now *"Proyecto 2000 regions"* and *"Proyecto de Salud y Nutrición Básica regions"*). Difficulties persist in the development and dissemination of a technical norm as several different protocols for the integrated management of child health have been developed. Also, each project has a large training component designed to disseminate the project's own protocols. No common indicators or agreed framework exist for the monitoring and evaluation of any of these activities. In the area of institutional development, studies have been duplicated (e.g. in health financing, information systems) without a channel for clearing terms of reference or drafts with the authorities. Not surprisingly, these studies led to no decision and to no action.

Duplication is underpinned by a fragmented budget system. The treasury finances some of the fixed costs (labor costs, MINSA's large pension payments for retirees-included in MINSA's budget, and some goods and services). Discretionary expenditures are financed by "projects" and by revenues from tariffs. These resources are managed separately from the funds provided by the treasury and are spent according to different rules and often by different decision-makers. Each project reports loosely to the MINSA Office of International Financing, Investment, and Cooperation (OFICE) and to the Ministry of Economy and Finance (MEF) through the MINSA Office of General Planning (OGP). Two separate units in MEF monitor the health projects. One for *Salud Básica* and another for the projects financed with foreign loans. No public agency has aggregated information about the financial flows or progress indicators of the projects financed by bilateral donors (some of which are large).

MINSA has begun to tackle some of these issues through the creation of a "Public Sector Modernization Coordination Unit (UCM)". This unit, headed by a team of strong technicians, has begun to assign priorities and eliminate duplications in the area of institutional development. At the time of writing, little action had been taken to improve institutional responsibilities for MCH and environmental health.

WEAKNESS OF THE INFORMATION SYSTEMS

The weakness of the information on health service production in Peru is striking and past attempts to correct this have lacked continuity and consistency. While other countries in LAC would worry about problems of measurement of 10-20%, in Peru estimates of the production of key health services vary by 200%. For 1995, estimates of the production of ambulatory consultations range from 30 to 68 million for the sector as a whole. Much of the variation in estimates comes from ignorance about private sector production, but the data concerning direct provision of services by MINSA is not much better. Estimates for ambulatory consultations run from 15 million (official statistics) to 27 million (household survey estimates) for 1995. There is inconsistent reporting of non-clinical services produced (e.g. for health education, extramural consultations), and for other non-clinical services that are measured (e.g. vector control activities, laboratory production). There is no attempt to consolidate the data or to produce it in a way that allows for comparisons. A similar problem exists with the measurement of inputs for MINSA. The data is poor even for expensive items such as staff, training, or the provision of equipment, since each program or funding source maintains its own records and there is neither a human resources nor infrastructure office in MINSA to consolidate such information. Official immunization data (perhaps the best official data available) indicate significantly higher coverage than survey data (e.g. a 10% difference for tuberculosis vaccination).

The problem arises from a combination of factors that include failure to use the information that is available, duplication, and the existence of incentives not to provide the information.

Lack of use: At the national level, the MINSA Office of Statistics and Information (OEI) is responsible for collecting and compiling data, and produces annual statistics and reports that are typically published with a lag of several years. No office or agency is in charge of reviewing or further analyzing the data on a regular basis. The situation is similar at the regional level. Although a few regions have produced special studies (usually associated with special requests for funding), this is the exception, as they are not required to report on anything that goes beyond the proof of compliance with financial procedures. There also seems to be little use of information at the local level where personnel may lack the skills needed for data interpretation. The few areas where there have been attempts to use data as the basis for regular supervision and feedback have opted for the use of parallel information systems.

Duplication: Providers spend large amounts of time and resources filling duplicate forms to report on similar subjects to different authorities, and the more forms there are to fill up, the more the quality of all of them is watered down. In addition to reporting to the Health Information System (HIS) and to the epidemiological surveillance system, most providers report to six or more vertical programs and often to one or more projects, donors or NGOs (no agency trusts the other agency's data –usually with good reason). This duplication has reached the point where providers see it as a serious burden.

Incentives to report: In some areas, providers have incentives to hide information, such as reporting activities that produce revenues from tariffs or information revealing low levels of productivity or short hours of work. Programs with high political visibility and concomitant high coverage goals, such as the family planning program, also provide incentives for over-reporting.

Most MINSA providers today report to the Health Information System (HIS), developed in the late 1980s with assistance from a USAID-financed project. The HIS data is usually produced and summarized on paper by the provider, centralized at the local level, entered into electronic files at the Departmental level and compiled and managed in Lima. The whole process is the responsibility of MINSA's Statistics Office, which is also responsible for obtaining and compiling data from other public and private providers. This system is in critical condition: the most recent data published is for 1992. Data for 1993 and 1994 have been abandoned and the statistics for 1995, which tend to be used in most internal documents, are still under revision and are thought to suffer from serious inconsistencies. For example, family planning data have been found in at least one regional hospital to be seriously over-reported. HIS produces only outpatient data. While some hospitals in Lima send data to MINSA regularly, there is no system for compiling statistics for inpatient services —those used are for 1995 and come from the 1996 Infrastructure Census, an exercise that is not carried out regularly.[42]

There have been numerous attempts to develop information systems. Some of these systems failed before being fully developed, such as attempts to develop complex hospital cost accounting systems. Others were successful over the brief period when they responded to a perceived emergency such as the cholera epidemic of the early 1990s, or remain successful during a period when they receive special funding. These include vertical national programs such as family planning, or externally funded projects. In recent years, there have been several attempts to design proposals to overhaul the information system. Large and costly reports have been prepared by consultant firms financed by the projects, but have received scant attention from the authorities. Officials today are skeptical about wholesale reforms and tend to believe that the proposed blueprints may be technically good, but do not adequately address the institutional context of the sector.

The experience acquired with *Salud Básica* may point to a partial solution to some of these problems. Its funding from MEF has been accompanied by stringent demands of accountability which required timely data on financial management, on staff and on the production achieved by the establishments supported by the program. For the production data, PSBPT has created a national data base that uses selected information extracted from the sheets filled by the establishments to report to the HIS. This data is now available with a lag of less than two months for most of the establishments covered by *Salud Básica*. The program has done four things that need to be underscored. First, as the program funds some (or all) of the staff in the establishment, it is well placed to apply pressure for the timely compliance with its reporting requirements. Second, it circumvents the Ministry's slow regional data entering procedures by hiring a regional data entering technician, whose pay is related to timeliness in reporting. Third, it has created software with flexible, user-friendly features that allows it to produce the regular reports required by MEF (though other types or formats of analyses, if desired, are very cumbersome to extract). Fourth, although more incipient, the production of these statistics and their review has initiated an interesting dialogue between the center, which is now in a position to identify problems, and the regions. In 1997, the program requested that all regions produce justification and remedies for all providers with production levels lower than certain benchmarks. This justification was made a condition for the renewal of contracts, and hence generated considerable interest. Clearly, a consideration for the future is that once the data are effectively used for evaluation or for payment, there is a need to establish auditing procedures and accountability for misrepresentation.

While the geographical coverage achieved by *Salud Básica* is high, the amount of information collected is small. It is limited to the number of services delivered, classified as either intramural, extramural, or preventive/promotional. Increasing the usefulness of these data for specific MCH program monitoring will require adjustments to the current

---

[42] Most of the "production statistics" used in this report are from household surveys and not from administrative sources.

system. Expanding the *Salud Básica* system to replace the HIS will be challenging and it will require a strong effort by the authorities to be selective to avoid overburdening the system.

The reforms being implemented in Peru's health system, as it shifts in response to the priority challenge of reducing inequality in health care, thus require new skills at every level. The next chapter, on "Human Resources in Health Care", looks at the new training, and new incentives, needed if the right kind of health professionals with an appropriate skills mix are to be found, in the right locations, and in sufficient numbers.

7. HUMAN RESOURCES FOR HEALTH CARE

Human resource issues are at the root of many inefficiencies and inequities in the Peruvian health system. This chapter focuses on issues of human resource quality, skills mix, and geographical distribution that have a bearing on the impact of health services for the poor. As background for the discussion, the trends in the labor market are discussed.

THE LABOR MARKET FOR HEALTH PROFESSIONALS

Labor market indicators point to an excess supply of health professionals in recent years. This glut has developed a buyers market and has been used by employers to circumvent some of the large benefits mandated by the "*Ley Médica*" approved by the government to appease a doctors' strike in 1989-90. MINSA has been taking advantage of this market situation to impose short term contract hiring on a large scale. These contracts run for three months—though it is now proposed to extend them to one year—and carry none of the social benefits received under regular forms of employment, viz. medical or disability insurance, pension, vacations, and severance pay. All *Salud Básica* doctors are employed under such contracts, but also those hired to fill slots opened by departing physicians in hospitals and other regular MINSA jobs. IPSS has also benefited from the labor market situation, but in a different way. For close to a decade IPSS has steadily reduced the number of medical professionals hired under regular public sector employment contracts. Using a mix of termination incentives, salary cuts (in real terms), and outright dismissals justified under a 1990 institutional "rationalization" decree, it has succeeded in transferring a large part of its staff to private personal service employment contracts, which provide less security of tenure and fewer social benefits. Thus, the largest IPSS hospital (Almenara) halved its staff from 4,000 to 2,000 over 1990-91, but almost immediately began to re-employ workers under service contracts.

There has been some debate in Peru about the origin of the labor market glut. The *Federación Médica* (the physicians' union) and the *Colegio Médico* (the Professional Association) think it has arisen from a large increase in the supply of new professionals graduating from several new medical schools and are calling for "restraint" in the training of additional professionals. These organizations document their concern explaining that the number of doctors licensed to practice by the *Colegio Médico*, grew about 5% in 1997, significantly faster than the population.[43]

However, a long-term review of market trends shows that the number of health sector professionals working in Peru has grown only moderately during the last 15 years. The

---

[43] Colegio statistics are not exact, despite a requirement that all practicing physicians be re-licensed in 1997. Pre-1997 Colegio figures overestimate the total because of unreported deaths (though most are reported to collect burial benefits), retirements, dropouts from the profession, and emigration. On the other hand, the post re-licensing figures of 1997 underestimate the total because several thousand registered and practicing physicians did not re-license. To correct for the latter omission CUANTO carried out a 1% sample of the 4,472 registered members who had not re-licensed and found that 71% of that number were indeed still practicing. The resulting estimate is that there were approximately 25,500 practicing physicians in 1997. New licenses granted during 1997 totaled 1,392, a 5.5% increase. However, the net increase in the stock is less by an unknown amount— CUANTO estimates between 4.7 to 5.0 percent--given retirements, deaths etc. during the year (Webb 1998).

supply has begun to expand more rapidly only in recent years. The increase in the number of medical schools did not significantly increase the total supply of students because San Fernando (the largest medical school) significantly reduced its intake of medical students during the years of economic stagnation. A review of the long-term trends in the market suggests that the glut is more readily explained as an effect of the collapse in public and private spending during the economic crisis of 1988-1993, rather than as a result of growth in the rate of graduation. It also suggests that the current glut may be temporary as the ratio of physicians per inhabitant –which grew from 0.5 per thousand inhabitants in 1964, to 0.7 in 1980 and to 1.0 in 1997– remains low by international standards when adjusted for income per capita. This is consistent with the low fraction of GDP assigned to the health sector in Peru (see Chapter 1). Because of this low initial level, demand for health services can be expected to grow rapidly as income grows and health services become available to new segments of the population. The increase in the number of non-physician health sector workers over the last three decades has been roughly similar to that of physicians. The ratio of non-physicians to physicians has remained at about 3 to 1 over that period.[44]

GEOGRAPHICAL INEQUALITY

A standing indictment of health provision in Peru has been geographical inequality and, above all, an extreme concentration of medical resources in Metropolitan Lima, and, by contrast, an extreme deficit in the more backward Sierra and Amazon rural areas of Peru. In 1964, the availability of physicians was 5 times higher in Lima than in the rest of the country. Things have improved since then, as the per capita availability of physicians in Lima over that period rose by 37 percent while in the rest of Peru it rose 124 percent. Availability today is generally good throughout the Coast (80 percent of all physicians, 52 percent of the population). Even the Sierra has improved substantially (17 percent of physicians, 35 percent of the population).[45] Much of the improvement was brought about by urban growth outside Lima, which provided a natural pull for physicians. Part of it, however, was achieved through government intervention and specifically as a result of two programs: SERUM and the *Salud Básica*.

The SERUM program, created in 1982, superseded an earlier program, which required all medical students to work without pay for a year in rural or urban low-income neighborhood health establishments as a condition for graduation. SERUM is not a requisite for graduation, but is a requirement for employment in the public health sector and for admission to government internship programs for further specialization.[46] As the number of applicants is larger than the paid positions available, applicants compete for

---

[44] 1964 data from Hall [1969], Table 2-12, p. 62. 1996 and 1997 data from (Webb 1998) below, and from INEI*Encuesta Nacional de Hogares* (ENAHO). Other sources seem less reliable. The 1996 "*II Censo Nacional de Infraestructura yRecursos Humanos de Salud*" is not corrected for duplication caused by multiple job-holding nor for undercounting of professionals working in private practice offices. Thus, the Census counted 2,622 dentists—far below the 6,960 estimated by ENAHO and the 9,000 dentists registered by the *Colegio Odontologico del Peru*. A published May 1986, "ANSSA-Peru.*Analisis del Sector Salud. Recursos Humanos del Sector Salud del Perú. Informe Técnico No. 5*" uses 1981 Census figures and a more detailed 1985 sample survey to study the geographical distribution of health workers, but non-physician occupational categories are not well-defined and major categories are omitted.
[45] The contrast is much larger if it is borne in mind that distances are much shorter and transportation much cheaper on the coast than in the Sierra (highlands).
[46] This transition from compulsory unpaid to voluntary paid programs was common in several LAC countries during the transition to elected governments that took place in the 1980s.

paid positions, which receive the starting government salary for physicians. Many applicants who do not manage to obtain a paid position then join the program without pay as a means to gain experience and the possibility of a public sector job in the future. SERUM has expanded markedly since its inception, from 272 in 1983 to 804 in 1990, and to 1,107 in 1997; the number of *serumista* nurses rose from 400 to 500 in the same period.

Since 1994, the *Salud Básica* Program finances salaries and bonuses for health staff in rural and urban low-income locations. The financial incentives used are large. Whereas bonuses for remote locations in countries such as Bolivia or Honduras are in the order of 15% and are available only for selected areas (usually international frontiers) and for selected types of professional, Peru has taken a radical approach. Bonuses are paid on a gradient that depends on the difficulty of the location and can be as much as 200% of the total salary of a comparable government worker. PSBPT pays staff in two ways. Some are government employees who benefit from a second payment to extend their hours of service. Others are not public employees, and are hired on temporary contracts which are periodically renewed –these staff often receive higher salaries than the regular employees, but have no benefits and no security in the job. Over 10,000 staff work in this manner. Of them, 15% are physicians, 35% are other professionals and 50% are health technicians (e.g. auxiliary nurses). This program today finances 40% of the MINSA physicians in the poorest seven departments and 17% of MINSA physicians nationally.

Despite the effort to improve geographical distribution, persistent inequality is likely to remain a major obstacle to health improvement in Peru over the medium, and even long run. Despite the salary bonus paid to physicians who agree to work in public health establishments located in the least accessible and poorest areas, turnover in those positions is exceedingly high. Consensus opinion in MINSA is that higher salaries will not overcome the combined effect of the pull of professional careers, tied to city-based medical specialization and private practice, and the burden of life in a radically different cultural environment deprived, moreover, of the customary "needs" of urban living. One effect of those negative incentives is reflected, as already noted, in short stays and so high turnover rates in the more distant and impoverished regions. *Salud Básica* physicians average about two years of service before beginning residence to obtain a specialization. But the turnover problem is in fact greater than is suggested by that two-year statistic, because even during that period, physicians find ways to obtain transfers and to move, step-wise, from the most distant, to less distant rural establishments, then to small urban establishments, and finally to cities. *Serumistas* follow a similar process even during their short, one-year service. Evidence of this process is provided by the statistical correlation between years since graduation and distance from urban centers. As a result, large and exceedingly poor population groups in rural areas of the Sierra (highlands) and Selva (Amazon jungle) are unlikely to see a significantly greater availability of trained physicians for the foreseeable future.

This conundrum is leading specialists to look for alternative solutions to the problem of serving rural communities. An option under discussion would involve a change in the skills-mix for the local health workers complemented with stronger links to the rest of the health network. Local workers would be more in charge of the public health aspect of the job with less emphasis on the clinical aspects. The systems of communications and reference would need to be strengthened, and in some areas the use of mobile physicians and "telehealth technology" would be introduced.

QUALITY OF TRAINING

Consensus among MINSA officials and medical professional leaders is that standards in medical education have been falling. This is mostly associated with the recent large-scale and little regulated creation of new university faculties in medicine. Many of these are located in provincial cities that have almost no resource base for meeting the human and physical teaching requirements of a modern medical education. At the same time there is a continuing multiplication in the number of teaching institutes for non-physician medical workers. Universities must obtain licenses, but permissions to operate have been granted liberally in recent years and, once in operation, universities need no further governmental or professional approval to grant professional titles to physicians. The licensing of non-university teaching centers is not subject to professional approval or certification. According to the president of the *Federación Médica*, medical malpractice suits are on the rise.

It is more difficult to arrive at a judgment on standards with respect to nursing education. The last two decades have seen two major changes in that schooling. During the mid-1980s, nursing education was converted from what was essentially an intermediate-level, technical training into a "professional", university-level education. Schooling requirements rose from three to five years and educational establishments were required to affiliate with a university. Teaching content became more bookish and less practice-based, while the strong "warmth and service" orientation of nursing schools—commonly run by religious groups—gave way to a more career (professional quality) orientation. Paradoxically, the longer, five-year study period was often not full-time, so that effective study-time may have become shorter. The second change in nursing education has consisted of a multiplication in the number and variety of teaching centers, both "professional" or university-level programs, and shorter, non-degree programs. Opinions on the overall effect of these changes are mixed. On the whole, the nurse is thought to be better trained for primary care, including rural and community health service, than is the physician. One question, however, is whether a standardized "nurse" is an appropriate product. Hospitals and clinics demand division of labor and so specialization. Rural service demands different, and probably less specialized skills.

MISMATCH BETWEEN SKILLS-MIX AND NEEDS

The mismatch takes two forms. One is that the content of medical training has not kept up with the shift in national priorities toward primary and preventive health, or with the corresponding shift to community and rural health delivery models. The educational gap is in part a matter of the relative attention given to different medical pathologies, and partly of non-medical knowledge and skills related to public health and to community work. At the same time the training of medical professionals has not kept up with the rapidly increasing importance of systems, teamwork and information in health delivery, and therefore, with the need for administrative and managerial skills. The educational system is beginning to respond to these gaps. Medical faculties in universities are creating public health departments and courses, while non-university educational centers in both management and medical fields are creating programs in both public health and medical administration. San Fernando, which remains the largest medical faculty, has recently opened a strong, public health management program, competing directly with ESAN, and has also strengthened its program in reproductive health. But additional efforts will be needed to close these gaps.

The other mismatch has to do with the mix and appropriateness of medical professionals for poor rural communities, the hard core of the poverty-related health problem. Despite an impressive and expensive expansion in rural primary health delivery over the last three to four years, mortality and morbidity rates remain high while the frequency of professional consultations remains low. The effectiveness of physicians in these rural health establishments, especially in carrying out communal and preventive health tasks and dealing with environmental health risks, is reduced by high turnover rates. Behind that turnover lie deep cultural and socioeconomic gaps, and also powerful professional incentives. On grounds of both cost and effectiveness, therefore, it is difficult to be optimistic about the odds of achieving a significant further extension of health care to the rural poor with the current, standard physician. Unfortunately, there seems to be no consensus within the health sector in Peru regarding the solution to this problem.

Obstetrices (midwives) have university-level training to attend the reproductive health needs of women, and are health professionals trained parallel to nurses, unlike most other countries where nurse-midwifery is a postgraduate specialization for nurses. There are many fewer *obstetrices* than nurses in Peru, and they have always been clustered in urban hospital settings. Under *Salud Básica*, they have become better distributed among rural facilities, along with physicians. The professional conflict between *obstetrices* and nurses has kept nurses from playing more of a role in maternal health care, to the detriment of many health services where there is no *obstretriz* on staff. The priorization of maternal and perinatal health care for reduction of maternal and perinatal mortality will require that nurses (and health technicians in many cases) obtain the proper necessary training to provide that care in underserved areas. With malnutrition being a major problem for maternal and child health, nutritionists are in very short supply –only 1800 are registered with the *Colegio de Nutricionistas*, and of those, 40% work in public sector jobs, mostly in urban areas. Most nutritionists are not prepared for public health nutrition. They tend to be clinical or laboratory dieticians. Training in nutrition for physicians and *obstetrices* is also very limited: all nurses are trained in child growth and development. Some university schools of medicine, nursing and midwifery have added breastfeeding to their curricula in recent years.

8. CONCLUSIONS AND RECOMMENDATIONS FOR A REFORM AGENDA FOCUSING ON THE POOR

This chapter presents recommendations regarding the development of a reform agenda directed to improving the health status of the poor. It begins by summarizing the main conclusions about health priorities and goes on to discuss recommendations in four areas: provision, financing, reorganization of MINSA, and human resource policy.[47]

HEALTH PRIORITIES

While much of the population enjoys a health status similar to that of the Latin American average, and while there have been important gains in the health of the poor in recent years, there exists a marked gap between the health outcomes for the poor and the non-poor. Reducing that gap requires sustained emphasis on primary health, accompanied by a greater emphasis on the needs of poor mothers and young infants and by better efforts to control communicable diseases. Looking into the near future, there is also a need to initiate implementation of preventive measures and screening for early detection of chronic diseases.

To continue to improve the health status of mothers and young infants, there is a need to increase the coverage and quality of Safe Motherhood interventions. To achieve this, in addition to strengthening services in primary clinics, two changes are necessary. First, interventions will need to go beyond the primary clinic level, strengthening obstetric services at the secondary level, and developing effective communications, transportation and reference systems. Several options should be pursued to achieve this, including expanding the use of private providers (who are already important suppliers of these services). Second, in addition to strengthening the supply of these services, it is crucial to expand the use of these services by the poor. This requires moving into a population-based system with measurable targets for key interventions (such as the coverage of births by skilled personnel). It also requires policies to help the poor overcome the cost barrier.

The poor suffer to a larger extent than the rest of the population from the reemergence of communicable diseases. There is a need to increase the effort and efficiency in the management of these diseases. This may require assigning more resources to this area. It also requires moving beyond the one-size-fits-all model of primary services. Given the great regional diversity that characterizes Peru, combating these diseases in a more effective way requires greater flexibility in the use of resources and greater local capacity for implementation. In many cases, the local capacity of the health authorities can be greatly enhanced by greater community participation. The prevention of many diseases

---

[47] The fragmentation of the health sector of Peru calls for reform. Other countries are striving to increase efficiency in their health sector by introducing market-based reforms that reduce fragmentation and introduce competition in health services. Lessons from those experiences make it clear that these reforms require a long period of implementation. Peru should consider embarking on such a major reform, but it cannot afford to wait until the benefits of such a reform reach the poor. The next logical step would be to continue to build on the important reforms of recent years in order to have an immediate impact on the health of the poor.

and poor health conditions requires multi-sectoral interventions at the regional and local level, covering water and sanitation, education and agriculture. These interventions are difficult to organize and the capacity to enter into inter-sectoral interventions needs to be strengthened. There is also a need for a stronger national epidemiological surveillance system to increase the capacity to respond with specialized support to control outbreaks. Also needed is a health information system that is capable of providing useful data to monitor the priority programs more frequently than the five-year interval that is now possible with the ENDES surveys.

REFORMS IN THE PROVISION OF SERVICES

The report identified the need for changes in targeting; improved access of the poor to hospital services; and higher quality and more efficient delivery of primary care by the public sector.

The most important action in relation to the targeted programs is to take measures to *reduce their vulnerability to fiscal or political crises*. The cut in fiscal spending in 1998 was mainly concentrated in the targeted programs. While the rest of the system is permanent and politically powerful, the targeted programs have ad hoc arrangements such as short term contracts and could easily be dismantled or modified.

Targeting can be strengthened by introducing internal improvements to the programs that are already targeted and by making external reforms to target the rest of the provision of care. Internally, there is scope to increase the accuracy of the targeting both across and within regions: (i) The accuracy of the methodology to target across regions is blunted by the existence of other objectives in guiding the allocation of funds, such as occupation of frontier areas, and these other objectives should be funded separately to avoid loss of transparency on the methods of targeting; (ii) Most regions have poor and less poor areas within them. As there exist many forces that tend to pull resources towards the better-off areas, a periodic audit of the specific location of the programs within regions should be implemented; and (iii) Improved poverty maps using more powerful analytic techniques and taking advantage of modern software could be incorporated to the planning tools in use by the programs. This should be done with care to minimize the loss of the transparency and simplicity that characterized the old poverty maps.

The main benefits of improved targeting would derive from external reforms to incorporate more programs into the targeting framework and unify that framework. All programs should be planned as part of a wider of public expenditure effort, rather than individually. As transfers are used to compensate for regional shortfalls in financing, MINSA should make an effort to identify regional expenditures from all public sector programs, including those of high relevance to health that are managed by other agencies. Much could be achieved by going beyond the special programs and improving the distribution of the "core budget" – which is currently mainly assigned to hospitals. This would require improving the geographic distribution of these resources and improving the use of hospital facilities by the poor.

Every effort should be made to increase the access to hospitals by the poor. A minimum amount of hospital resources should be assigned for the treatment of the poor. This will be difficult to achieve as there exists no foolproof way to identify the poor, but it is urgent to initiate pilots on different ways to achieve it. A pilot could require that hospitals increase their production of birth deliveries and basic surgery (it is only the poor who are not getting these services today). Another could use systematic data and procedures to screen those patients who request exemptions —this will be particularly useful for patients requiring costly elective interventions or chronic treatment. The government should also consider piloting community insurance schemes for catastrophic health problems.

A policy needs to be developed linking any future large scale investment program for hospitals with needed reforms. The policy should clarify the "mission" of public hospitals, improve the financial incentives for hospitals, develop a regulatory capacity and establish interventions to increase hospital services for the poor. The "mission" should include the provision of secondary-level services to the poor and some level of insurance against catastrophic events to the uninsured. The priorities for the specific services to be provided should originate from the overall health priorities. As argued in Chapter 2, in the medium term these should emphasize the provision of obstetric, emergency and other basic surgery.

Incentives should be developed based on the progress already achieved towards autonomy. Financial incentives and independence should be strengthened, not restricted with bureaucratic red-tape. However, these incentives need to be made consistent with the public policy objective of financing hospital services. The most commercialized hospitals today receive two-thirds of their financing as lump sum transfers with no conditions or specified objectives attached to them (and they get to use the assets for free). The new system should attempt to link increasing fractions of the total financing with the desired outputs and to establish some competition among providers. Some hospitals, including many of the National Hospitals, may be ready to move to a corporatized system where the hospital becomes responsible for all of its costs, including the payroll, and where the government would pay for services provided, and not for inputs. Other hospitals need to be given incentives to gear themselves to provide services that complement those offered by the primary clinics of an area, and some of the financing for the hospital could be channeled through those clinics. To increase efficiency, competition should be a key component of the framework. The development of competition requires that hospital services financed by the government are also purchased from IPSS providers and from the private sector; it also requires that public hospitals be allowed to sell services to IPSS and private insurers.

MINSA never developed a regulatory capacity for hospitals and should attempt to do it in a limited way and avoiding as much as possible the use of bureaucratic controls. At minimum, three areas require regulation. First, hospitals should begin to report their activities, and should do it in a way that allows performance to be measured against objectives. Second, high-tech investments tend to have large economies of scale and to require high levels of utilization to be operated in a safe manner. These investments should be cleared by a body with oversight over MINSA and IPSS and should include the participation of the private sector.

To reform the provision of primary health care, it is essential to continue working with the CLAS and to carefully review the plans for *Redes*. The CLAS continue to be under attack by some public officials, but enjoy recognition by the communities. Specific recommendations at this point are:

- Establish mechanisms to monitor progress on the local health plans of CLAS;
- Develop units (possibly covering several regions) to provide technical assistance to the CLAS in the areas of organization, local health planning and evaluation, provision of services, community extension, multisectoral integrated community development, and other areas.
- Undertake permanent systematic evaluation of the CLAS program to monitor its impact on coverage, quality and opportunity of services, and community participation. The monitoring should include comparisons with other primary health clinics and should serve to make continual improvements in the system;
- Provide incentives and resources to allow some CLAS to expand their local health plans to include the management of environmental risks;
- Improve the institutional dialogue of MINSA and the CLAS. Strengthen the office that coordinates the CLAS so that proper support can be provided to CLAS at the local level. Replace the adversarial system of audits of CLAS, conducted by opponents to the system, with a more supportive system that will include the provision of technical assistance in the area of financial management.

While the concept of *Redes* is promising, it involves bureaucratic risks and could jeopardize the delicate and essential component of community participation as the principal administrative unit becomes farther removed. To avoid these risks:

- Establish clearly the role to be played by the health regions and subregions before creating new layers of bureaucracy to manage the *Redes*;
- Maintain the autonomy of CLAS by giving them funds to purchase goods and services from higher level facilities and allow them to voluntarily join networks (instead of making them part of *Redes* by administrative fiat);
- Encourage local experimentation. There are no best-practice blueprints that would recommend a top-down homogenous approach.

REFORMING THE FINANCING OF CARE

The direct and indirect costs of services have created an economic barrier for the poor. To confront this barrier, MINSA should pursue its work in the *Seguro Escolar* and the *Seguro Materno-Infantil*. The *Seguro Escolar* should be improved and simplified. First, reviewing the tariff levels and the tariff structures used for reimbursements to bring them in line with the full cost of services. Second, improving the logistics used for reimbursements by simplifying the paperwork and by reimbursing in cash. Even if this implies a loss in price gains associated with larger purchases, the loss would be balanced by a more timely availability of cash. Third, reviewing the impact of the scheme on the willingness of providers to work.

The *Seguro Materno Infantil* should become a priority. The plan should reimburse co-payments for services and the costs of drugs and medical inputs. Reimbursement rates should be set at levels sufficiently high to make key inpatient activities currently of difficult access for the poor (especially births and maternal complications) attractive for the providers. Reimbursements should also be designed in a way to create incentives for prevention, extramural activities and referrals. Incentives to the users should take into account indirect costs, such as transport and childcare. Lessons should be learned from experience acquired with the *Seguro Escolar* concerning reimbursement procedures. Bureaucratic procedures that could stifle the system should be avoided.

In the short run, the government has decided to implement the two schemes independently and to limit the choice of providers to MINSA facilities. In the medium term, and once the basic procedures have been tested in this logistically easier context, the two schemes should incorporate more developed features in two areas. A wider array of services could be covered if the non-poor contribute through the payment of insurance premiums. Second, competition and improved quality could be obtained by extending the choice of providers to include other public and private providers.

REORGANIZATION OF THE MINISTRY OF HEALTH

In the past there have been numerous attempts to implement sweeping reforms. Given the complexity of the issues, the resistance to change from many participants in the sector and the likely political cost of wholesale reforms, MINSA should take an incremental approach. The initial steps of reform should be chosen according to health priorities. Three specific recommendations are proposed below:

- First, continue to develop a think tank (based on the Public Sector Modernization Unit) to support the Authorities in the development and implementation of policy and in strengthening the planning function. The unit would: (i) provide support in the development of health priorities (objectives) based on the use of epidemiological studies and economic principles, ensure that these objectives are applied by the different programs, and translate the objectives into monitorable action plans that would serve as a basis for the formulation of the budget; (ii) use and disseminate health sector information, including periodic reports on the achievement of health priorities and annual estimates of National Health Accounts (NHA); and (iii) coordinate the different initiatives to separate financing from provision (described in Chapters 3 and 5).

- Second, develop a strategy for institutional reform geared to reducing duplication. This task would require three activities: (i) identification of all areas of unnecessary duplication within MINSA; (ii) development of a methodology to characterize needed change, including the mainstreaming of projects (clarifying definitions and principles, and identifying the cost of reform); and (iii) design of an Action Plan that would select areas for reform based on the expected cost-effectiveness of change.

- Third, develop information systems. MINSA should build incrementally on the HIS, based on the progress already achieved by *Salud Básica* and emphasizing the use of incentives to report. It is extremely important to establish that funds allocated will be increasingly based on the data provided and proven productivity. Use of the HIS system should be generalized to all programs and distinguish curative versus preventive and intramural versus extramural activities. The use of parallel systems should be progressively abolished and surveys and special studies should be used to collect complementary information without overburdening the HIS reporting sheet. Also it is urgent to create a reporting system for hospital inpatient services.

REFORMING HUMAN RESOURCE POLICIES

The government should sustain the efforts to improve the distribution of health workers and should introduce measures to improve the quality and skill mix in the health sector in a way that better serves the needs of the poor. Five specific recommendations are made to that effect:

- Review the employment terms in the public sector. It is unclear what effects are produced by the extraordinary degree of contractual dualism that exists in the public sector. This arrangement has costs: (i) The lack of security implied by short contracts is difficult to reconcile with the need for career public sector doctors. A degree of commitment seems required on each side to build up the particular types of knowledge and skills that go with public and primary health oriented work of the public sector physician; (ii) Most short term employees are currently concentrated in *Salud Básica*, while long term physicians work in hospitals, creating a vulnerability in primary care. *Salud Básica* would almost certainly be a first victim of any new budget cutbacks for health. At the other extreme, the current security of tenure is a major impediment to the plans for administrative reform. The Review of Employment Terms should also analyze the costs and benefits of maintaining SERUM and *Salud Básica* as separate programs.

- Establish a human resources department in the ministry of health. The sector lacks an administrative unit empowered to address sector-wide human resources issues. Such a unit should be created in the Ministry of Health and granted executive authority to set minimum personnel standards, as well as to determine procedures for hiring and periodically evaluating existing personnel. Its goal would be to ensure a high level of professional and personal competence as well as the best possible fit between the skills and training of sector professionals and the human resource needs determined by public health priorities.

In addition, the Human Resources Department would be responsible for all training of existing public health personnel. Training must become a continuous, sustained activity throughout the sector, and should therefore be the responsibility of a permanent, sector-wide authority which would thus become responsible for a multiplicity of training programs that are currently being carried out by different projects and programs. A particularly important responsibility would be to ensure the coordination and sustainability of the various programs that coexist in the attempt to upgrade peri-natal and maternal-infant capacity in public health establishments.

- Introduce a public medical service examination. As the dominant employer by far, and given the current glut in the labor market, the public sector (including IPSS) has the means to influence both standards and educational content through the entire system simply by setting high standards and defining the educational content required for public sector employment. The instrument that suggests itself most readily is a national level medical public service examination. [48] This would finesse the politically ticklish issue of a direct approach to the universities, and leaves considerable room for building legitimacy and for minimizing objections by bringing other institutional actors—above all the *Colegio*, the *Federación*, and two or three prestigious international teaching centers—into the process. Also, MINSA has the obligation and the means to raise the quality and the appropriate skill content of its own physicians.

It should be the Ministry's role to define standards and content for public sector employment. The principal "skill content" objective would be better preparation in community or public health, in management, and in primary care pathologies. The examination need not grade only one, all-purpose set of skills. It could also rate students on specialized topics that are in high demand by the government, such as management or rural health problems. The examination itself should perhaps be administered by the *Colegio* or some other independent, technical body. The involvement of an international prestige center, would perhaps confer an element of legitimacy. [49]

- Modify the mix of subsidies for medical specialization. The government currently spends approximately US$5 million annually for the medical specialization in residence in local hospitals of some 300 to 400 recently titled physicians. The fields of specialization should be modified to give greater emphasis to public health, community delivery, primary care pathologies, and health establishment administration. A start in this direction is already being made, with the allocation of 30 residencies to San Fernando for specialization in public health. Consideration should also be given to the inclusion of non-medical professionals and for "residence" in establishments other than hospitals, for instance, in a government planning or administrative office, or in a sequenced series of smaller health establishments.

- Introduce certification of university medical programs. The effort to upgrade and modify the content of physician training could be strengthened by direct pressure on

---

[48] Government market power is immense. About two out of three practicing physicians currently work in the public sector. In addition, most young physicians are likely to want to keep open the option of government employment, on a full or part time basis, even if their immediate career choice is full time in the private sector.

[49] Once established, an entrance examination could become a stepping stone to two further initiatives. It would provide a precedent for the periodic evaluation of all practicing physicians. Such an evaluation would have to be a *Colegio Médico* initiative and process, but MINSA could prompt and assist the *Colegio* in that direction. The entrance examination would also legitimize a second initiative—the periodic evaluation of all public sector physicians.

universities through a certification process. The process would necessarily have to be carried out by the _Colegio_, but MINSA should begin conversations with the _Colegio_ on this proposal and offer to support the initiative. The financing of a study of quality in medical teaching would perhaps be the first and most important form of support.

BIBLIOGRAPHY*

Altobelli, Laura C. 1998. "Comparative Analysis of Primary Health Care Facilities with Participation of Civil Society in Venezuela and Peru". Processed. Division of State and Civil Society (DPP/SCS) of the Inter-American Development Bank. Washington, D.C.

_____ 1998. "Health Reform, Community Participation, and Social Inclusion: The Shared Administration Program." UNICEF. Lima.

Alvarado, Betty, Gladys Garnica and María Elena Romero. 1996. "Análisis de Costos de los Servicios de Salud: Perú 1994." Informe de la Universidad del Pacífico. Ministerio de Salud. Lima

Banco Central de Reserva del Perú. 1998. *Estudios Económicos* (April). Lima.

Beaumont, Martín, Julio Gamero and María del Carmen Piazza. 1996. *Política Social y ONGs*. Lima: DESCO.

Castañeda, Tarsicio. 1998. "Como llegar a los Pobres con Programas de Salud en el Perú: Retos y Recomendaciones." Processed. World Bank. Washington, D.C.

Concha, Mari Sol. 1998. "Situación de Salud y Tendencias." Processed. World Bank. Washington, D.C.

_____ 1998. "Provisión de Salud." Processed. World Bank. Washington, D.C.

Cortez, Rafael. 1998. "Equidad y Calidad de los Servicios de Salud: El Caso de los CLAS." Informe de Consultoría de la Universidad del Pacifico. Ministerio de Salud. Lima.

Cortez, Rafael A, Arlette Beltrán and Mariella Bautista. 1996. "Análisis de la Demanda por Servicios de Salud: Peru 1995." Universidad del Pacífico. Lima.

Fernández Díaz, Jesús. 1997. "Revisión de Estudios de Financiación del Sistema de Salud del Perú. Implicaciones para el Proceso de Reforma del Sector." Ministerio de Salud. Lima.

Fiedler, John L. 1993. "The Organized, Private Health Care Market of Peru, 1980-1993." Report submitted to the Chief of the Office of Health, Population and Nutrition, USAID/Peru. Lima.

---

* The word processed describes informally reproduced works that may not be commonly available through libraries.

Francke, Pedro. 1998. "Lineamientos para una Política de Focalización del Gasto Público y Tarifas del Ministerio de Salud." First draft. Processed. Ministerio de Salud. Lima.

_____ 1997. "Una Propuesta para la Focalización del Gasto Público en Salud en el Perú." Processed. Ministerio de Salud. Lima.

_____ 1997. "Distribución del Subsidio Público en Salud por Quintiles, Perú 1994." Processed. Ministerio de Salud. Lima.

_____ 1997. "Exoneraciones y Tarifas en los Establecimientos del Ministerio de Salud." Processed. Ministerio de Salud. Lima.

_____ 1996. "Informe No. 1. Estratificación por Provincias para la Asignación de Gastos en Salud." Processed. Ministerio de Salud. Lima.

Frisancho, Ariel.1993. *Salud Comunitaria en el Ande Peruano. Reflexiones sobre una Experiencia de Cooperación con Médicos y Enfermeras en Servicio Rural.* Lima: Programa de Salud Comunitaria en el Trapecio Andino.

Gwatkin, Davidson. 1999. "Fact Sheets on Health, Nutrition, Population and Poverty in Peru." Processed. World Bank. Washington, D.C.

_____ 1998. "The Current State of Knowledge about Targeting Health Programs to Reach the Poor: Implications for World Bank Operations." Initial discussion draft. Washington, D.C.

Gwatkin, Davidson R. and Michael Guillot. 1998. "The Burden of Disease Among the Global Poor: Current Situation, Future Trends, and Implications for Research and Policy." Prepared for the Global Forum for Health Research. Washington, D.C.

Heras, Antonio. 1996. "Assistance to the Ministry of Health, Peru. Contract Design-Health Sector Reform Project of Department LA1 (Latin America)." London: Institute for Health Sector Development.

Harding, April and Alexander Preker. 1998. "Innovations in Health Care Delivery: Organizational Reform within the Public Sector." Processed. World Bank. Washington, D.C.

Iglesias, Arturo. 1993. "Valoración de Rendimiento de los Hospitales Públicos de Lima Metropolitana y Callao." Processed. Lima.

Inter-American Development Bank. 1995. "Challenge for Peace: Towards Sustainable Social Development in Peru." Washington, D.C.

Instituto Nacional de Estadística e Informática. 1997. *Perú: Encuesta Demográfica y de Salud Familiar 1996*. Co-published by Macro International Inc., Calverton, Maryland, USA

_____ 1992. *Perú: Encuesta Demográfica y de Salud Familiar 1991/1992*. Co-published by Asociación Benéfica PRISMA and Macro International Inc., Columbia, Maryland, USA.

Khoman, Sirilaksana. 1997. "Rural Health Care Financing in Thailand: Innovations in Health Care Financing." World Bank Discussion Paper 365. Washington, D.C.

MACROCONSULT S.A. 1996. "Análisis del Gasto Público en Salud." Processed. Ministerio de Salud. Lima.

Ministerio de Salud. 1999. Programa de Fortalecimiento de Servicios de Salud. "Propuesta de Implementación del Seguro Materno Infantil." Lima.

_____ 1998. Programa de Salud Básica para Todos. *Memoria 1994-1997*. Lima.

_____ Oficina General de Epidemiología. 1998a. "Situación de Salud y Tendencias: Definición de Prioridades." Lima.

_____ Oficina General de Epidemiología. 1998b. "Dinámica Demográfica del Cambio a la Continuidad." Lima.

_____ Oficina General de Epidemiología. 1998c. "Panorama de la Mortalidad en el Perú." Lima.

_____ 1998. Programa Administrativo de Acuerdo de Gestión. "Reunión Nacional de Administración Compartida". Lima.

_____ 1998. *Plan Operativo 1998-Programas Nacionales de Salud*. Lima.

_____ PAAG-PSBPT-PAC. 1998. *Los Comités Locales de Administración de Salud*. Lima.

_____ PAAG-PSBPT-PAC. 1998. *Los Comités Locales de Administración de Salud (CLAS): Guia I para Organización y Gestión de CLAS*. Lima.

_____ Programa de Administración de Acuerdos de Gestión. 1998. *Hacia la Equidad con Eficiencia y Calidad*. Lima.

_____ 1997. "Evaluación del Programa de Salud Básica para Todos 1996: Uso y Percepción de los Servicios de Salud por la Población Focalizada." Lima.

_____   1997. *Análisis del Financiamiento del Sector Salud.* Lima.

_____   1996. Programa Salud Básica para Todos. "Evaluación Nacional PSBPT 1996: Resumen Ejecutivo." Lima.

_____   1996. *Informe Técnico No 1: Análisis de la Información de Defunciones en el Perú.* Lima.

_____   1996. *Informe Técnico No 2. Fecundidad, Planificación Familiar y Salud Reproductiva en el Perú.* Lima.

_____   1996. *Informe Técnico No 3. Metodología de Estratificación.* Lima.

_____   1996. *Informe Técnico No 4. Resúmen Gráfico de la Situación de Salud del Perú.* Lima.

_____   /UNICEF. 1996. *Los Comités Locales de Administración.* Lima.

_____   Oficina de Estadística e Informática. 1996. *2do Censo de Infraestructura Sanitaria y Recursos del Sector Salud 1996.* Vol I. Lima.

Peñarrieta, Isabel. 1998. *"Evaluación de Resultados; Equidad según necesidades de atención y comportamiento de los usuarios entre servicios CLAS y no CLAS-Subregion Lima Norte."* Lima.

Pollit, Ernesto, Enrique Jacoby and Santiago Cueto. 1996. *Desayuno Escolar y Rendimiento.* Lima: Editorial Apoyo.

Ramírez Eslava, Walter. 1998. *Desarrollo e Implementación del SICI en el Hospital Victor Ramos Guardia de Huarás.* Ministerio de Salud. Lima.

Reyes, Carmen and Moisés Ventocilla. 1997. "Revisión y Actualización del Financiamiento del Sector Salud 1995-1996. Informe Final." Lima: Ministerio de Salud.

Suárez, Rubén. 1993. "Public and Private Expenditure in Health Services in Peru: 1980-1992." Processed. Washington, D.C.

Tamayo, Gonzalo, Pedro Franke, Andrés Medina, Elmer Cuba and Augusto Portocarrero. 1997. *Análisis del Gasto Público en Salud.* Ministerio de Salud. Lima.

The Development Group, Inc. 1991. *Peru Health Sector Assessment.* Virgina, VA.

USAID/Peru. 1997. "Addressing Threats of Emerging and Re-Emerging Infectious Diseases. (527-0391) VIGIA." Lima.

UNICEF. 1994. *El Mapa de la Inversión Social. Pobreza y Actuación de FONCODES a nivel Departamental y Provincial.* Lima.

Vásquez, Enrique H., Rafael Cortez, and Carlos Parodi. 1998. "La Iniciativa 20/20 y los Servicios Sociales Básicos en el Perú 1980-1997." Universidad del Pacífico. Lima.

Verdera, Francisco V. *Seguridad Social y Pobreza en el Perú: una aproximación.* Documento de trabajo No. 84. Instituto de Estudios Peruanos. Lima.

Waters, Hugh. 1998. "Productividad en los Proveedores de Servicios del Ministerio de Salud del Perú." Processed. Ministerio de Salud. Lima.

Webb, Richard. 1998. "Los Profesionales del Sector Salud: Problemas y Propuestas." Processed. World Bank. Washington, D.C.

_____ 1998. "Evaluación de Medio Término del Proyecto de Salud y Nutrición Básica: Relevancia, Contribución a la Reforma y Coordinación." Processed. World Bank. Washington, D.C.

World Bank. 1997. *Sector Strategy. Health, Nutrition and Population.* Washington, D.C.

_____ 1995. "Peru: Strategic Planning for Health Sector Reform." Report No. 13710-PE, Human Resources Division, Country Department III, Latin American and the Caribbean Region Office. Washington, D.C.

Zschock, Dieter K. 1986. "Health Sector Analysis of Peru: Summary and Recommendations." HSA-PERU Reports. Stony Brook, NY.